Competency-Based Critical Care

Series Editors

John Knighton, MBBS, MRCP, FRCA
Consultant
Intensive Care Medicine & Anaesthesia
Portsmouth Hospitals NHS Trust
Portsmouth
UK

Paul Sadler, MBChB, FRCA
Consultant
Critical Care Medicine & Anaesthesia
Queen Alexandra Hospital
Portsmouth
UK

Founding Editor

John SP Lumley
Emeritus Professor of Vascular Surgery
University of London
London
UK

and

Honorary Consultant Surgeon
Great Ormond Street Hospital for Children NHS Trust (GOSH)
London
UK

Other titles in this series

Sepsis
Simon Baudouin (Ed.)

Sara Blakeley (Ed.)

Renal Failure and Replacement Therapies

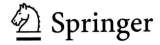 Springer

Sara Blakeley, BM, MRCP, EDIC
Queen Alexandra Hospital
Portsmouth
Hampshire, UK

British Library Cataloguing in Publication Data
Renal Failure and Replacement Therapies.—(Competency-based critical care)
   1. Kidneys—Diseases   2. Kidneys—Diseases—Treatment
   3. Acute renal failure   4. Acute renal failure—Treatment
   I. Blakeley, Sara
   616.6′1
   ISBN-13: 9781846289361

Library of Congress Control Number: 2007927934

Competency-Based Critical Care Series ISSN 1864-9998

ISBN: 978-1-84628-936-1   e-ISBN: 978-1-84628-937-8

9 8 7 6 5 4 3 2 1

springer.com

Contents

Contributors

Mohan Arkanath, MRCP
Consultant Nephrologist
Doncaster Royal Infirmary
Doncaster, UK

Sara Blakeley, BM, MRCP, EDIC
Queen Alexandra Hospital
Portsmouth
Hampshire, UK

Nerina Harley, MBBS, MD, PGDIPEcho,
    FRACP, FJFICM
Intensive Care Consultant
The Royal Melbourne Hospital
Victoria, Australia

Stephen Holt, PhD, FRCP
Consultant Nephrologist and Honorary
    Senior Lecturer
Sussex Kidney Unit
Brighton and Sussex University Hospitals
Royal Sussex County Hospital
Brighton, UK

Himangsu Gangopadhyay, MD, MBBS,
    FFARCS(Ireland), FJFICM
Consultant in Intensive Care
Frankston Hospital
Frankston, Victoria, Australia

Tim Leach, BM, FRCP
Consultant Nephrologist
Wessex Renal and Transplant Unit
Queen Alexandra Hospital
Portsmouth, UK

Emile Mohammed, MB, ChB, MRCP (UK)
Lecturer in Medicine (University of the West
    Indies) and Consultant Nephrologist

School of Clinical Medicine and Research
Queen Elizabeth Hospital & Cavehill Campus
Bridgetown, Barbados

Harn-Yih Ong
Registrar Intensive Care
St Vincent's Hospital
Melbourne, Victoria
Australia

Marlies Ostermann
Consultant Nephrology and Critical Care
Intensive Care Unit
St Thomas' Hospital
London, UK

John H. Reeves, MD, MBBS, FANZCA, FJFICM,
    EDIC
Consultant in Intensive Care and Anaesthetics
Department of Anaesthesia and Pain
    Management
Alfred Hospital
Melbourne, Victoria
Australia

Tom Sutherland, MBBS (Hons)
Radiology Registrar
St Vincent's Hospital
Melbourne, Victoria
Australia

Laurie Tomlinson, MRCP
Specialist Registrar Nephrology
Sussex Kidney Unit
Brighton and Sussex University Hospitals
Royal Sussex County Hospital
Brighton, UK

1
Assessment of Renal Function

Mohan Arkanath

Normal Functions of the Kidney

To be able to assess a degree of renal function or dysfunction, it is important to first consider the normal functions of the kidney:

1. *Maintenance of body composition:* The volume of fluid in the body, its osmolarity, electrolyte content, concentration, and acidity are all regulated by the kidney via variation in urine excretion of water and ions. Electrolytes regulated by changes in urinary excretion include sodium, potassium, chloride, calcium, magnesium, and phosphate.

2. *Excretion of metabolic end products and foreign substances*: The most notable are urea and a number of toxins and drugs.

3. *Production and secretion of enzymes and hormones:*
   a. Renin: See Figure 1.1.
   b. Erythropoietin: A glycosylated, 165-amino acid protein produced by renal cortical interstitial cells that stimulates maturation of erythrocytes in the bone marrow.
   c. 1, 25-Dihydroxyvitamin D_3: The most active form of vitamin D_3, it is formed by proximal tubule cells. This steroid hormone plays an important role in the regulation of body calcium and phosphate balance.

The Role of the Kidney in Homeostasis

Maintenance of body fluid composition and volume are important for many functions of the body. For example, cardiac output and blood pressure are dependent on optimum plasma volume, and most enzymes function best in narrow ranges of pH or ion concentration.

The kidneys take up the role of correcting any alterations in the composition and volume of body fluids that occur as a consequence of food intake, metabolism, environmental factors, and exercise. In healthy individuals, these corrections occur in a matter of hours, and body fluid volume and the concentration of most ions return to normal set points. In many disease states, however, these regulatory processes are disturbed, resulting in persistent deviations in body fluid volume and composition.

Body Fluid Composition

A large proportion of the human body is composed of water (Table 1.1). Adipose tissue is low in water content and, hence, obese individuals have a lower body water fraction than lean individuals. Because of slightly greater fat content, women generally contain less water than men.

Clinical Evaluation of Renal Function

Glomerular filtration rate (GFR) is generally considered the best measure of renal function; it is the sum of filtration rates of all of the functioning nephrons. It is defined as the renal clearance of a particular substance from plasma, and is expressed as the volume of plasma that can be completely cleared of that substance in a unit of time. In the following sections, we will compare the advantages

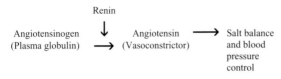

Figure 1.1. Production and secretion of enzymes and hormones for renin.

and disadvantages of the various methods available for GFR estimation or quantification.

$$\text{Clearance} \atop (\text{mL/min}) = \frac{\text{Urine}_x\,(\text{mg/dL}) \times \text{Volume}\,(\text{mL/min})}{\text{Plasma}_x\,(\text{mg/dL})}$$

Where x is the substance being cleared.

Features of an ideal marker for GFR determination:

- Appears endogenously in the plasma at a constant rate
- Is freely filtered by the glomerulus
- Does not undergo reabsorption or secretion by the renal tubule
- Is not eliminated by extrarenal routes

Urea

Urea was first isolated in 1773, and urea clearance as a surrogate marker for GFR introduced in 1929. Although urea measurement is performed frequently, it is well recognized that its many drawbacks make it a poor measure of renal function (see Table 1.2). For example, the rate of production is influenced by factors such as the availability of nitrogenous substrates, and the rate of reabsorption in the tubules can be affected by volume status.

Table 1.1. Body fluid compartment volumes[a]

	Example for a 60-kg patient
TBW = 60% × body weight	60% × 60 kg = 36 L
ICW = ⅔ TBW	⅔ × 36 L = 24 L
ECW = ⅓ TBW	⅓ × 36 L = 12 L
Plasma water = ¼ ECW	¼ × 12 L = 3 L
Blood volume = Plasma water ÷ (1 − hematocrit)	3 L ÷ (1 − 0.40) = 6.6 L

[a]TBW, total body water; ICW, intracellular water; ECW, extracellular water.

Table 1.2. Other factors altering blood urea or serum creatinine[a]

	Increased level	Decreased level
Urea	Prenatal causes (e.g., congestive heart failure, volume contraction) lead to increased tubular reabsorption • Gastrointestinal bleeding • Catabolic state • Corticosteroids • Hyperalimentation • Tetracyclines	Cirrhosis Protein malnutrition Water excess (e.g., SIADH, saline infusion) leads to reduced tubular reabsorption
Creatinine	Overproduction (e.g., rhabdomyolysis, vigorous sustained exercise, anabolic steroids, dietary supplements such as creatine) Blocked tubular secretion (e.g., drugs such as trimethoprim and cimetidine) Assay interference (e.g., ketosis and drugs such as cephalosporins, flucytosine, methyldopa, levodopa, and ascorbic acid)	Decreased muscle mass

[a]SIADH, syndrome of inappropriate ADH secretion.

Creatinine

Creatinine is a metabolite of creatine and phosphocreatine found in skeletal muscle. It is a small molecule that is not protein bound and, hence, freely filtered by the glomerulus. It does, however, undergo tubular secretion which is variable (see Table 1.2). Creatinine production can vary in an individual over time with muscle mass changes or acutely with massive myocyte turnover. There are also age- and sex-associated differences in serum creatinine (S_α) concentration; it is lower in the elderly and in women.

The ratio between *serum* urea and creatinine can be useful when assessing the patient with acute renal failure. Under normal circumstances, the ratio between urea and creatinine is 10:1 but this value can rise to greater than 20:1 when the extracellular volume is contracted. A volume-contracted state (*prerenal*) is a "sodium avid" state and promotes proximal tubular and distal nephron reabsorption of urea but not creatinine. Acute tubular necrosis (ATN) will have a urea-to-creatinine ratio of 10:1 because tubular reabsorption of urea is not preferentially increased.

Assessment of GFR

S_α has become a standard measure of renal function because of its convenience and low costs; however, it is crude marker of GFR. A 24-hour creatinine clearance (C_α) is often used in practice as a measure of the GFR because creatinine is freely filtered and not reabsorbed by the tubule. However, approximately 15% of urinary creatinine is a result of tubular secretion and, thus, this method overestimates GFR. The other problems with C_α are incomplete urine collection and increasing creatinine secretion. Inulin clearance is traditionally considered the "gold standard" for the measurement of GFR (1). It is one of the most accurate measures of renal function, but the inconvenience of administration, cost, and limited supply of inulin preclude its use in routine practice.

Estimated C_α: The Cockroft and Gault Formula (2)

This formula is used to estimate C_α at the bedside using age of the patient and S_α value (both correlate inversely with GFR), and the ideal body weight (IBW) of the patient.

This formula can used only when the S_α value is in a steady state and not when it is rapidly changing, as in acute renal failure. It has also been shown that S_α and estimations of GFR using various formulae are often inaccurate in critically ill patients (3). Although they may give an *estimate*, their limitations should be remembered when assessing renal function in patients on the intensive care unit. Other factors, such as urine output, clearance of acid and electrolytes, and rate of change of serum urea and creatinine should all be considered together.

The Cockroft and Gault formula is:

$$\text{Estimated } C_\alpha = \frac{(140 - \text{patient age}) \times (\text{weight in kg})}{(S_\alpha \text{ in } \mu\text{mol/L})}$$

Multiply by 0.85 for women, 1.23 if male.

Urinalysis (4, 5)

The microscopic examination of the urinary sediment is an indispensable part of the work-up of patients with renal insufficiency, proteinuria, hematuria, urinary tract infections, or kidney stones. A careful urinalysis has been referred to as a "poor man's renal biopsy." The urine should be collected as a midstream catch or fresh catheter specimen, and because the urine sediment can degenerate with time, it should be examined soon after collection. Urinalysis should include a dipstick examination for specific gravity, pH, protein, hemoglobin, glucose, ketones, nitrites, and leucocytes. This should be followed by microscopic examination if there are positive findings. Microscopic examination should check for all formed elements: crystals, cells, casts, and infecting organisms.

Appearance

Normal urine is clear, with a faint yellow tinge caused by the presence of urochromes. As it becomes more concentrated, its color deepens. Bilirubin, other pathologic metabolites, and a variety of drugs may discolor the urine or change its smell.

Specific Gravity

The urine specific gravity is a conveniently determined but inaccurate surrogate of osmolality. Specific gravities of 1.001 to 1.035 correspond to an osmolality range of 50 to 1000 mOsm/kg. A specific gravity near 1.010 connotes isosthenuria (urine osmolality matching plasma).

The specific gravity is used to determine whether the urine is, or can be, concentrated. During a solute diuresis accompanying hyperglycemia, diuretic therapy, or relief of obstruction, the urine is isosthenuric. In contrast, with a water diuresis caused by overhydration or diabetes insipidus, the specific gravity is low. It is also useful in differentiating between prerenal cause of renal failure (high) and ATN.

Volume

In health, the volume of urine passed is primarily determined by diet and fluid intake. The minimum amount passed to stay in fluid balance is determined by the amount of solute being excreted (mainly urea and electrolytes), and the concentrating ability of the kidneys. In disease, impairment of concentrating ability requires increased volumes of urine to be passed for the same solute output.

- *Oliguria* is defined as the excretion of less than 300 mL/d of urine, and is often caused by intrinsic renal disease or obstructive uropathy.
- *Anuria* suggests urinary tract obstruction until proven otherwise.
- *Polyuria* is a persistent, large increase in urine output, usually associated with nocturia. Polyuria is a result of excessive intake of water (e.g., compulsive water drinking), increased excretion of solute (hyperglycemia and glycosuria), a defective renal concentrating ability, or failure of production of antidiuretic hormone (ADH).

Chemical Testing

Blood

Hematuria may be macroscopic or microscopic (Table 1.3). Currently used dipstick tests for blood are very sensitive, being positive if two or more red cells are visible under the high-power field (HPF) of a light microscope. A disadvantage is that dipstick testing cannot distinguish between blood and free hemoglobin. A positive dipstick has to be followed by microscopy of fresh urine to confirm the presence of red cells and to exclude rare conditions such as hemoglobinuria and myoglobinuria. In female patients, it is essential to enquire whether the patient is menstruating.

Abnormal numbers of erythrocytes in the urine may arise from anywhere from the glomerular capillaries to the tip of the distal urethra. Dysmorphic erythrocytes tend strongly to be associated with a glomerular source. Abnormal proteinuria along with dysmorphic erythrocytes is a reliable sign of glomerular disease. Urinary tract abnormalities lead to microscopic or macroscopic hematuria but the erythrocytes exhibit normal morphology.

Protein

Proteinuria is one the most common signs of renal disease (Table 1.4). Most reagent strips detect a

TABLE 1.3. Causes of hematuria[a]

Glomerular disease	Mesangial IgA nephropathy
	Thin basement membrane disease
	Mesangial proliferative GN
	Membranoproliferative GN
	Crescentic GN
	Systemic lupus erythematosus
	Post streptococcal GN
	Infective endocarditis
	Alport's syndrome
Vascular and tubulointerstitial disease	Acute hypersensitivity interstitial nephritis
	Tumors (renal cell carcinoma, Wilm's tumor, leukemia)
	Polycystic kidney disease
	Malignant hypertension
	Analgesic nephropathy
	Diabetes mellitus
	Obstructive uropathy
Urinary tract diseases	Carcinoma (renal pelvis, ureter, bladder, urethra, prostate)
	Calculi
	Retroperitoneal fibrosis
	Tuberculosis
	Cystitis
	Drugs (e.g., cyclophosphamide)
	Trauma
	Benign prostatic hypertrophy
	Urethritis
	Platelet defects (e.g., idiopathic or drug induced thrombocytopenic purpura)

[a]GN, glomerulonephritis.

concentration of 150 mg/L or more in urine. They react primarily to albumin and are insensitive to globulin or Bence-Jones protein. False-positive results are common with iodinated contrast agents; hence, urine testing should be repeated after 24 hours. The normal rate of excretion of protein in urine is 80 ± 24 mg/24 h in healthy individuals, but protein excretion rates are somewhat higher in children, adolescents, and in pregnancy. Fever, severe exercise, and the acute infusion of hyperoncotic solutions or certain pressor agents (e.g., angiotensin II or norepinephrine) may transiently cause abnormal protein excretion in normal individuals.

The protein in normal and abnormal urine is derived from three sources:

1. Plasma proteins filtered at the glomerulus and escaping proximal tubular reabsorption.
2. Proteins normally secreted by renal tubules.

TABLE 1.4. Causes of proteinuria based on pathophysiologic mechanism[a]

Glomerular proteinuria	Primary glomerular disease • Minimal change disease • Mesangial proliferative GN • Focal and segmental glomerulosclerosis (FSGS) • Membranous GN • Mesangiocapillary GN • Fibrillary GN • Crescentic GN	Secondary glomerular disease • Drugs: e.g., mercurials, gold compounds, heroin, penicillamine, probenecid, captopril, lithium, NSAID • Allergens: bee sting, pollen, milk • Infections: bacterial, viral, protozoal, fungal, helminthic • Neoplastic: solid tumors, leukemia • Multisystem: SLE, Henoch-Schonlein purpura, amyloidosis • Heredofamilial: diabetes mellitus, congenital nephritic syndrome, Fabry's disease, Alport's syndrome • Others: febrile proteinuria, postexercise proteinuria, benign orthostatic proteinuria
Tubular proteinuria	Endogenous toxins: light chain damage to proximal tubular, lysozyme (leukemia) Exogenous toxins and drugs: mercury, lead, cadmium, outdated tetracycline	
Tubulointerstitial disease	SLE Acute hypersensitivity interstitial nephritis Acute bacterial pyelonephritis Obstructive uropathy Chronic interstitial nephritis	
Overflow proteinuria	Multiple myeloma Light chain disease Amyloidosis Hemoglobinuria Myoglobinuria Certain colonic or pancreatic carcinomas	
Tissue proteinuria	Acute inflammation of urinary tract Uroepithelial tumors	

[a]GN, glomerulonephritis; NSAID, nonsteroidal anti-inflammatory drugs; SLE, systemic lupus erythematosus.

3. Proteins derived from the lower urinary tract or leaking into the urine as a result of tissue injury or inflammation.

Most patients with persistent proteinuria should undergo a quantitative measurement of protein excretion, with a 24-hour urine measurement. A protein excretion rate greater than 3.5 g/d (nephrotic range proteinuria) should prompt further investigations to ascertain the exact cause of the proteinuria with measurements of urea, creatinine, liver function tests (most importantly, serum albumin), and a full blood count. A definitive diagnosis has to be achieved with a renal biopsy. Nephrotic syndrome is defined as a combination of proteinuria in excess of 3 g/d, hypoalbuminemia, edema, and hyperlipidemia.

Glucose

Renal glycosuria is uncommon and any positive test requires evaluation of diabetes mellitus.

Bacteriuria

Dipsticks detect nitrites produced from the reduction of urinary nitrate by bacteria and also leucocyte esterase, an enzyme specific for neutrophils. Detection of both nitrites and leucocytes on dipstick has a high predictive value for urinary tract infection.

Urine Microscopy

An *un*spun sample of urine may be examined under low- or high-power microscopy, however, a *spun* sample is a more accurate. Urine is centrifuged, the supernatant is discarded, and an aliquot of the residue is placed on a glass slide using a Pasteur pipet. All patients suspected of having renal disease should have urine microscopy.

White Blood Cells

The presence of 10 or more white blood cells per cubic millimeter is abnormal and indicates an inflammatory reaction within the urinary tract. Most commonly this represents a urinary tract infection but it may also be found with a sterile sample in patients on antibiotic therapy, or with kidney stones, tubulointerstitial nephritis, papillary necrosis, or tuberculosis.

Red Blood Cells

As mentioned previously, erythrocytes can find their way into the urine from any source between the glomerulus to the urethral meatus. The presence of more than two to three red blood cells per HPF is usually pathological. Erythrocytes originating in the renal parenchyma are dysmorphic, whereas those originating in the collecting system retain their uniform biconcave shape.

Casts

Based on their shape and origin, casts are appropriately named. Hyaline casts are found in concentrated urine, during febrile illnesses, after strenuous exercise, and with diuretic therapy. They are not indicative of renal disease. Red cell casts indicate acute glomerulonephritis. White cell casts indicate infection or inflammation, and are seen in pyelonephritis and interstitial nephritis. Renal tubular casts are found in cases of ATN and interstitial nephritis. Coarse granular casts are nonspecific and represent the degeneration of a cast with a cellular element. Finally, broad waxy casts are indicative of stasis in the collecting tubules and are seen in chronic renal failure.

References

1. Brown SC, O'Reilly PH. Iohexol clearance for the determination of glomerular filtration rate in clinical practice: evidence for a new gold standard. *J Urol.* 1991; 146(3): 675–679.
2. Cockroft DW, Gault MH. Prediction of creatinine clearance from serum creatinine. *Nephron.* 1976; 16: 31–41.
3. Hoste EA, Damen J, Vanholder RC, et al. Assessment of renal function in recently admitted critically ill patients with normal serum creatinine. *Nephrol Dial Transplant.* 2005; 20(4): 747–753.
4. Henry JB, Lauzon RB, Schaumann GB. *Basic examination of the urine.* Clinical Diagnosis and Management by Laboratory Methods. 19th ed. Philadelphia: Saunders. 1991.
5. Graff L. A Handbook of Routine Urinalysis. Philadelphia: Lippincott. 1983.

Suggested Reading

Davison AM, Cameron S, Grunfeld J-P, et al. Oxford Textbook of Clinical Nephrology. 3rd ed. Oxford: Oxford University Press. 2005.

Greenberg A, Cheung AK, Coffman TM, et al. Primer on Kidney Diseases. 3rd Ed. London: Academic Press. 2001.

Guyton AC. Textbook of Physiology. 8th Ed. New York: Saunders. 1991.

2
Imaging of Acute Renal Failure—A Problem-Solving Approach for Intensive Care Unit Physicians

Tom Sutherland

Acute renal failure (ARF) is a common problem in hospitalized patients. It has a variety of causes, traditionally divided into prerenal, renal, and postrenal. A further classification can be made into medical and surgical causes, with the later defined as patients who will benefit from mechanical intervention.

Acute tubular necrosis (ATN) is the most common cause of ARF (approximately 45%) and postrenal obstruction accounts for roughly 10% of presentations (1). A variety of imaging modalities may be used to help diagnose the cause, or, if this is not possible, to differentiate medical from surgical causes. ARF in renal transplants will not be addressed.

Acute or Chronic Renal Failure?

This is best answered by clinical assessment rather than with imaging. Imaging findings in chronic renal failure are nonspecific and essentially characterized by small kidneys. X-rays can show the renal outline, calcification, renal bone disease and effects of hyperparathyroidism. Ultrasound is an excellent modality for structural imaging because it is able to detect reduced renal parenchyma, scarring (usually secondary to previous reflux nephropathy), calcification, and polycystic kidneys. The echogenicity of the cortex can be assessed with a hyperechoic cortex (normal cortex is hypoechoic to liver), present in most causes of chronic renal failure; adult polycystic kidney disease being the notable exception. Noncontrast computed tomographic (CT) and magnetic resonance imaging

(MRI) scans analyze renal structure and renal artery calcification, and dynamic gadolinium-enhanced MRI renal studies allow functional assessment. Other functional studies, such as mercaptoacetyltriglycine (MAG3) and diethylene triamine pentaacetic acid (DTPA) show reduced renal uptake and delayed excretion of tracer.

A further role of imaging is to determine the number of present and functioning kidneys. For ARF to occur in previously normal kidneys, the underlying cause must be a bilateral process, or else a single functioning kidney must be compromised (Figure 2.1).

Acute Tubular Necrosis

Ultrasound will usually show enlarged kidneys with a smooth contour caused by interstitial edema, no hydronephrosis, and renal arterial and venous flow. The examination of choice in suspected ATN is a MAG3 nuclear medicine study.

Scintigraphic examinations in ATN using Tc-99m-MAG3 demonstrate relatively well-preserved on-time renal perfusion, and delayed tracer uptake, often with a continuing activity accumulation curve. If the activity curve does have a maximum, the time to maximum is delayed (2). Excretion of tracer into the collecting system is delayed and reduced, but there is no obstruction to drainage of the collecting systems. If excretion and drainage occur, the time from maximal activity to half-maximal activity (or another quantitative measure of tracer excretion) is prolonged. What underlies this scintigraphic pattern

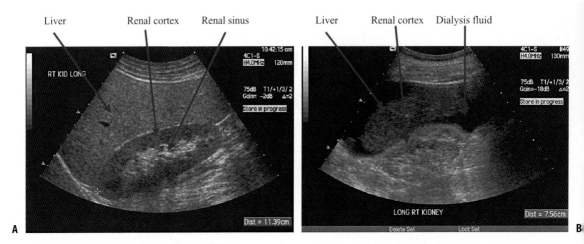

Liver   Renal cortex   Renal sinus   Liver   Renal cortex   Dialysis fluid

FIGURE 2.1. *A*, ultrasound of a normal kidney. Smooth cortex, hypoechoic to liver. *B*, chronic renal failure with a small irregular kidney with hyperechoic cortex compared with liver (anechoic area around the liver is peritoneal dialysis fluid).

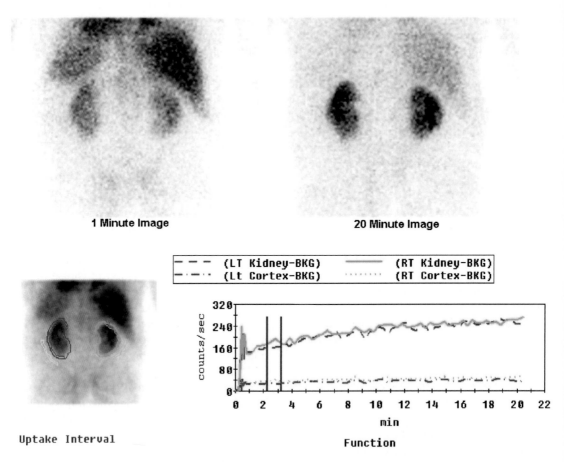

1 Minute Image   20 Minute Image

Uptake Interval   Function

FIGURE 2.2. MAG3 study showing progressive accumulation of tracer in the renal cortex indicating normal perfusion but no excretion, consistent with ATN. A normal activity curve should initially peak as the kidneys are perfused and then activity declines as tracer is excreted and passes into the bladder. Lt, left; Rt, right; Bkg, background.

is parenchymal retention of MAG3 by the remaining viable tubular cells, whereas tubular obstruction prevents drainage of tracer into the collecting system. The tubular cells continue to take up tracer while they are viable and, thus, the cortical activity can be used to monitor disease progress, with progressive loss of cortical activity being a poor prognostic indicator (Figure 2.2).

If a MAG3 study cannot be performed, ultrasound will demonstrate a cortex of normal echogenicity with either a normal or hypoechoic medulla. The renal arteries can also be interrogated for the renal index (RI), which is an objective measure of the resistance to renal perfusion. RI is defined as (systolic velocity minus diastolic velocity) divided by systolic velocity, and has been heavily investigated to determine whether elevation in RI can differentiate ATN from renal hypoperfusion not yet complicated by ATN. Unfortunately, there have been mixed results and, generally, RI has inadequate specificity for routine clinical use.

Glomerulonephritis and Acute Interstitial Nephritis

Clinical history and urinalysis plays a vital role in differentiating GN and acute interstitial nephritis (AIN) with the "gold standard" diagnostic test being a renal biopsy. The main role of imaging is to detect structural signs of chronic renal disease and to exclude other causes of ARF. MAG3 studies will show poorly functioning kidneys, but no accumulation pattern and also no obstruction to drainage. Edema can sometimes be demonstrated with ultrasound, manifest as hypoechoic large kidneys. If there is a clinical suspicion to direct imaging, a careful search may also find other signs of the underlying cause, for example, pulmonary hemorrhage in Goodpasture's syndrome and pulmonary nodules in Wegener's granulomatosis.

Ureteric Obstruction

For obstruction to produce ARF it must be bilateral or affecting a single functioning kidney. This is the classical cause of surgical ARF.

Ultrasound is the first-line test for obstruction. It is radiation free, portable, is not nephrotoxic, and can simultaneously gather other structural information. Obstructed kidneys are typically normal sized with dilated ureters, renal pelvis, and calyceal systems. These urine-filled structures appear as anechoic areas with posterior acoustic enhancement. Caution is required in interpretation because a ureter and renal pelvis may be dilated without being obstructed (a false positive). This can occur after previous obstruction that leaves a residual "baggy" collecting system, or as an anatomical variant (enlarged extrarenal pelvis). Differentiation can often be made by examining the bladder for ureteric jets, which are the periodic expulsion of urine from the ureter into the bladder, which can be detected by Doppler imaging. If ureteric jets are present, then there is not a complete obstruction on that side (3). False negatives can occur in the hyperacute setting if the renal collecting system has not had time to dilate, or if the system has spontaneously decompressed by forniceal or renal pelvis rupture (Figure 2.3).

Noncontrast CT scan is the gold standard for detecting ureteric calculi (4). The ureters can usually be traced between the kidney and bladder, and a hyperdense stone can be seen at the distal site of hydroureter. More than 99% of renal calculi are radiopaque on CT scan, however, xanthine calculi may be radiolucent and stones associated with indinavir are radiolucent. The obstructed kidney is typically edematous (i.e., swollen) with

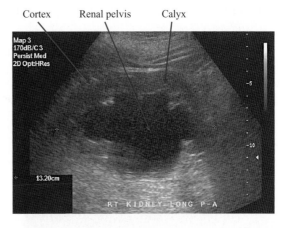

Cortex   Renal pelvis   Calyx

FIGURE 2.3. Ultrasound of a hydronephrotic kidney. Size is normal with dilated renal pelvis and calyces (the anechoic central part).

perirenal stranding. The administration of contrast is contraindicated in ARF because of its potential nephrotoxicity. Although not as helpful as a contrast-enhanced CT scanning, a noncontrast study can usually detect many extrinsic compressing masses, such as retroperitoneal tumors, or cervical or colon carcinomas, that may produce bilateral obstruction. Complications related to trauma, such as urinoma or renal pedicle avulsions, are also visible even without contrast (Figure 2.4).

Scintigraphic imaging with either Tc-99m-MAG3 or Tc-99m-DTPA can detect ureteric obstruction by showing a dilated collecting system with delayed drainage of tracer. The collecting system is outlined down to the level of the obstruction with no or limited tracer draining beyond this. The negative predictive value of nuclear medicine scanning is extremely high, with a normal study virtually excluding obstruction. Of course, sufficient tracer must be present in the collecting system to reach the obstruction point. Reduced urine production associated with renal failure may deliver so little tracer into the collecting system that obstruction cannot be excluded. The lower the patients glomerular filtration rate (GFR), the higher the probability of having an indeterminate study (5). Further, an enlarged but nonobstructed collecting system may mimic delayed drainage. In this latter situation, the specificity of the examination is increased by administering 20 mg (or sometimes 40 mg) of frusemide IV, and scanning for a further 20 minutes. A baggy nonobstructed system will promptly wash out, and the delay in washout after frusemide correlates with the degree of obstruction. Once again, it must be stressed that the only way mechanical obstruction can produce ARF in previously normal kidneys is by affecting a solitary functioning kidney, or by blocking both kidneys simultaneously.

Renal Artery Dissection or Occlusion

Each kidney is normally supplied by a single renal artery that arises from the aorta before dividing into an average of five segmental end-arterial branches. Arterial dissection and occlusion is another surgical cause of ARF. Renal infarction may be caused by blunt trauma with avulsion of the renal pedicle or penetrating trauma transecting the renal artery. Renal artery dissection may be iatrogenic, occurring during endovascular intervention. Bilateral dissection or exclusion from the circulation can occur secondary to an aortic dissection. Suspicion of a dissection or occlusion is virtually the only differential diagnosis that warrants the administration of intravenous CT contrast in the setting of ARF in which MRI scanning is unavailable. An arterial phase CT scan highlights the renal artery anatomy, demonstrating the intimal flap of dissection and can also detect signs of renal infarction and lacerations (6) (Figure 2.5).

Magnetic resonance angiography (MRA) has excellent sensitivity and specificity for detecting dissection and occlusion of proximal renal arteries. Segmental arteries are less well visualized, however, unilateral or isolated segmental pathology will not produce ARF. MR contrast is much

Arrow heads are fatty stranding.   Right ureteric calculus   Inferior pole left kidney

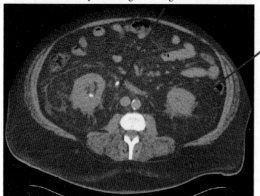

FIGURE 2.4. Noncontrast CT scan with complete right-sided and moderate left-sided obstruction secondary to bilateral ureteric calculi (left calculus not shown). Edematous fatty stranding around each kidney with the right calculus in the dilated ureter. *Arrowheads* indicate fatty stranding.

4
Acute Kidney Injury

Sara Blakeley

Patients may be admitted to the intensive care unit (ICU) with acute kidney injury (AKI) or it may develop during their stay. This chapter gives an overview of the definition and epidemiology of AKI, along with clinical features and initial investigations.

Definition of AKI

AKI is an abrupt (<7 d) and sustained decrease in kidney function (1). It is accompanied by changes in blood biochemistry (e.g., a rise in serum creatinine), in urine output, or both. There is a spectrum ranging from a mild transient rise in serum creatinine, to overt renal failure needing renal replacement therapy (RRT); hence, the term acute kidney injury (AKI) is more precise than the term "acute renal failure".

Multiple definitions of ARF exist, and the reader is guided to a series of excellent reviews that highlight this problem (1–5). A rise in serum creatinine is often used as a marker of renal dysfunction, but it is affected by extrarenal factors, such as age, sex, race, and muscle bulk. It may lag behind changes in glomerular filtration rate (GFR), either in decline or during recovery, and, therefore, does not always give a true reflection of the GFR. Urine output can be used to define renal failure, but this can be confounded by the use of diuretics, and not all cases of renal failure are associated with oliguria.

Efforts have been made to develop a universal and practical way of defining AKI via either serum creatinine or urine output. One such recent proposal is the RIFLE (5) system; an acronym for three levels of renal dysfunction and two renal outcomes. The levels of renal dysfunction can be defined by changes in serum creatinine, GFR, or urine output.

Risk of Renal Dysfunction
- Serum creatinine increased 1.5 fold *or*
- GFR decreased by more than 25% *or*
- Less than 0.5 mL/kg/h of urine for 6 hours

Injury to the Kidney
- Serum creatinine doubled *or*
- GFR decreased greater than 50% *or*
- Less than 0.5 mL/kg/h of urine for 12 hours

Failure of Kidney Function
- Serum creatinine increased 3 fold *or*
- An acute rise in creatinine of greater than 44 µmol/L so that new creatinine is greater than 350 µmol/L *or*
- GFR decreased more than 75% *or*
- Less than 0.3 mL/kg/h of urine for 24 hours or anuria for 12 hours
- *Note:* This takes into consideration acute-on-chronic renal failure

Loss of Kidney Function
- Complete loss of kidney function for longer than 4 weeks

End-Stage Renal Disease
- The need for dialysis for longer than 3 months

Incidence and Outcome

AKI develops in 5 to 7% of hospitalized patients (6, 7). Six to 25% of patients on the ICU develop AKI (2, 8); overall, 4% of admissions require RRT.

This may underestimate the scale of the problem, however, because when all degrees of kidney dysfunction are considered using the RIFLE criteria, 20% (9) of hospital patients and 67% of ICU patients developed some form of kidney injury (10).

The incidence and progression of AKI varies depending on the patient group studied. For example, up to 20% of cardiac surgery patients will develop some evidence of renal injury (11), but only 1% will need RRT (12).

AKI on the ICU is associated with a hospital mortality of 13 to 80% (2, 8, 10–17) and 57 to 80% if RRT is needed. Renal failure rarely occurs on its own, with up to 80% of patients with renal failure on the ICU having another organ system failure (8). Various factors have been associated with a worse outcome; including comorbidity, increased severity of illness, presence of sepsis, need for mechanical ventilation, oliguria, hospitalization before ICU, and delayed occurrence of AKI (13–15).

The development of AKI dramatically increases mortality across all patient populations studied (8–10, 12, 14). Worsening levels of renal dysfunction, as described by the RIFLE criteria, correlate well with increasing hospital mortality, with up to a 10-fold risk of death with "failure." AKI carries an independent risk of death, but it is unclear whether this is related to the systemic effects of renal failure itself, the effects of its treatment, or is simply a reflection of the severity of the underlying condition.

After AKI needing RRT, 10 to 32% of patients are discharged from hospital still needing RRT (2, 16, 18).

Causes of AKI

Causes of AKI can be divided into prerenal, intrinsic, and obstructive causes. One disease may be associated with different causes of ARF, for example, sepsis is a common cause of renal dysfunction on the ICU, accounting for up to 50% of cases of AKI. AKI occurs in 23% of patients with severe sepsis, and in 51% of patients with septic shock when blood cultures are positive (19). Sepsis is characterized by systemic vasodilation (*prere-*

nal failure) but intrarenal vasoconstriction, which could progress to tubular damage (*intrinsic* renal failure). Glomerular microthrombi are associated with disseminated intravascular coagulation, and can cause intrinsic AKI (20).

Prerenal Failure

Prerenal failure (Figure 4.1) accounts for 15 to 20% of cases of AKI on the ICU (13, 15). For the kidneys to be perfused and, therefore, function, adequate pressure, flow, volume, and patent vessels are needed.

The kidney autoregulates to maintain a constant renal blood flow (RBF) through a mean arterial pressure range of 65 to 180 mmHg. "Prerenal failure" is an appropriate, albeit exaggerated, physiological response to renal hypoperfusion. Stimulation of the renin-angiotensin-aldosterone system attempts to retain salt and water and, therefore, maintain RBF. Because renal tissue is still preserved, once renal perfusion is restored, function should improve. A profound or prolonged reduction in perfusion can, however, lead to ischemic acute tubular necrosis (ATN) (intrinsic renal failure).

Conditions leading to reduced renal perfusion and, therefore, causing prerenal failure are:

- Hypotension (relative or absolute) secondary to vasodilation (e.g., certain drugs, loss of vascular tone, and sepsis)
- Compromised cardiac function
- Intravascular volume depletion (absolute or effective)
- Increased intra-abdominal pressure (abdominal compartment syndrome)

Intrinsic Renal Failure

The commonest cause of intrinsic renal failure on the ICU is ischemic ATN developing after profound or prolonged prerenal failure (Figure 4.2). Up to 80% of cases of AKI on the ICU are attributed to ATN (2, 13, 15). Although ATN is a histological diagnosis, its development is suggested by the persistence of renal failure following the restoration of adequate renal perfusion. The

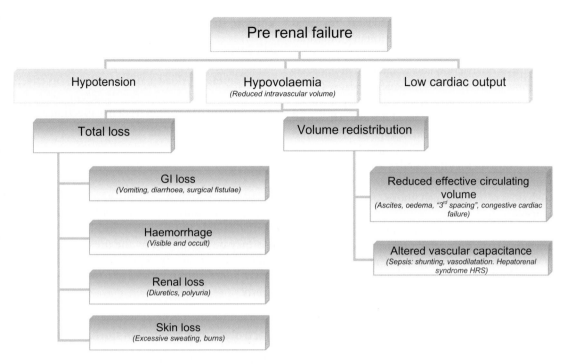

Figure 4.1. Causes of prerenal failure. GI, gastrointestinal.

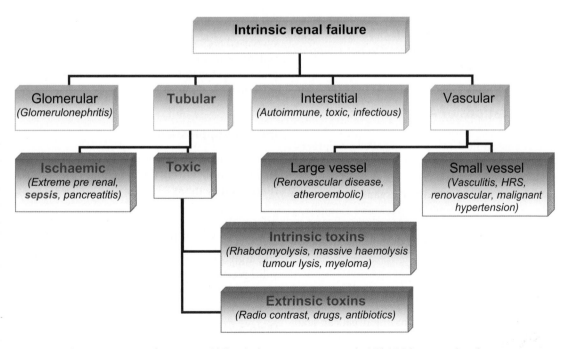

Figure 4.2. Causes of intrinsic renal failure (*red*, commoner causes on the ICU). HRS, hepatorenal syndrome.

pathophysiology of ischemic ATN is reviewed elsewhere (21, 22), but an alteration in glomerular hemodynamics with marked afferent arteriolar renal vasoconstriction causes a fall in glomerular filtration pressure and subsequently causes ischemia. This particularly affects the outer medulla. Tubular damage leads to loss of normal cell-to-cell adhesion and allows back leakage of filtrate into the interstitium. Shed cells precipitate, with protein obstructing the tubules and further compromising tubular function. Local inflammatory mediators respond to cell injury, perpetuating the process.

ATN can also develop secondary to a variety of intrinsic or extrinsic renal toxins. Vascular causes of renal failure may be present at a prerenal or intrarenal level, and should be considered in vasculopaths. The more classic glomerular causes for intrinsic renal failure are seen less frequently on the ICU, but are important to recognize because they require specific treatment.

Postrenal or Obstructive Renal Failure

Obstruction can occur at any level of the urinary collecting system and can be caused by intrinsic (e.g., stones, tumor) or extrinsic causes (e.g., surrounding or infiltrating tumor, large inflammatory abdominal aortic aneurysms). Obstruction is an infrequent cause of AKI on the ICU but is important to be excluded in all cases.

Complications of AKI

AKI is a systemic disease, having effects on practically all organ systems (23). It is becoming increasingly recognized that there is "cross talk" between the injured kidney and other organs through the release of proinflammatory cytokines. Complications related to other failing organs may be seen, but complications specific to the failing kidney are as follows.

Retention of Uremic Toxins

Accumulation of toxins, including urea, can lead to nausea, vomiting, drowsiness, a bleeding tendency, uremic flap, and, rarely, coma (uremic encephalopathy) and a pericardial rub.

Volume Overload

Salt and water retention occurs early, and is a common reason for initiating RRT on the ICU (16). Volume overload may have deleterious effects on cardiac and respiratory function, with the development of peripheral edema affecting wound healing and pressure areas.

Acidosis

There is retention of organic anions (e.g., phosphate) and reduced production of bicarbonate by the failing tubules. In critically ill patients, this may be aggravated by the presence of a nonrenal acidosis, for example, lactic acidosis from sepsis and respiratory acidosis from respiratory failure.

Electrolyte and Mineral Disturbances

Hyponatremia, hyperkalemia, and hyperphosphatemia are commonly seen.

Anemia

Anemia can develop because of inappropriate levels of erythropoietin (decreased synthesis) or increased red cell fragility, causing premature red cell destruction. Uremia is also associated with platelet dysfunction and increased risk of gastrointestinal bleeding.

Immunosuppression

Renal failure itself can impair humoral and cellular immunity, putting the patient at risk of infectious complications.

Metabolic Consequences

Hyperglycemia occurs because of peripheral insulin resistance and increased hepatic gluconeogenesis. Protein catabolism is also activated.

Drug Accumulation

Renal failure may be secondary to drugs, but, as GFR falls, renal clearance of drugs and their

TABLE 5.1. Risk factors for ARF

Risk factor	Selected reference(s)
Older age	Nash et al., 2002 (43)
Diabetes	Parfrey et al., 1989 (44).
Underlying renal insufficiency	
Cardiac failure	
Sepsis	Brun-Buisson et al., 2004 (45)
	Ricci et al., (46)
Absolute or relative hypovolemia	
Hepatic failure	Han and Hyzy, 2006 (47)
Nephrotoxins (including	Barrett et al., 1993 (48)
high-osmolality	Aspelin et al., 2003 (49).
radiocontrast agents)	McCullogh et al., 2006 (50)
Cardiopulmonary bypass with	Mangano et al., 1998 (51)
aortic cross-clamping	Chertow et al., 1998 (52)
(particularly valve surgery)	
Nonrenal organ transplantation	Lima et al., 2003 (53)
Abdominal compartment syndrome	McNelis et al., 2003 (54)

treatments such as diuretics. Urine volume is of little diagnostic value, although little or no output is acutely useful with causes of anuria, including shock, bilateral urinary obstruction, renal cortical necrosis, and bilateral vascular occlusion.

Other Markers of Renal Injury

These have been described but are not currently generally available in the acute setting. For example, serum cystatin C has been recently proposed as a marker of ARF (4), predicting ARF by at least 24 hours.

Radiology

Renal ultrasound is the modality of choice to exclude obstruction. Reduced renal size and cortical thinning (although preserved in diabetic nephropathy) is indicative of chronic renal impairment. A helical computed tomographic (CT) scan may be useful in urolithiasis, but there are risks of secondary injury with radiocontrast.

Renal Biopsy

Renal biopsy is considered when noninvasive evaluation has not established the diagnosis (5); the major indications include isolated hematuria with proteinuria, nephrotic syndrome, acute nephritic syndrome, and unexplained ARF. Percutaneous biopsy is most commonly performed and the

inherent risks of bleeding should be weighed up in the setting of the risk-to-benefit ratio.

Note: The "gold standard" for the diagnosis of a prerenal cause of ARF is resolution of renal impairment in response to fluid challenge. This is in contrast to significant ATN, in which there is prolonged time to resolution.

Primary Prevention

Primary prevention of ARF in the critically ill with or without baseline risk factors consists of avoidance, amelioration, and treatment of these factors wherever possible. Strategies can be divided into nonpharmacological, for example, fluid administration to reduce the risk of contrast induced nephropathy (6), and pharmacological. To date, no pharmacological strategies have conclusively demonstrated prevention of ARF from any insult (7).

Loop Diuretics

Although oliguria (<400 mL/24 h) is common in ATN, anuria is rare and other etiologies must be considered. Nonoliguric patients have a better prognosis than oliguric patients in terms of a greater residual GFR (8), lower peak serum creatinine, and dialysis-free survival at 21 days (9, 10), possibly reflecting less severe renal injury. A clinical issue of the use of loop diuretics often arises in increasing the urine output of oliguric patients.

Experimentally, loop diuretics reduce active sodium chloride transport in the thick ascending limb of the loop of Henle, decreasing energy requirements and, thus, protecting the cell in the setting of decreased energy availability. Only anecdotal human evidence suggests that the use of loop diuretics may be beneficial in the first 24 hours in flushing tubular casts. There is no evidence of benefit in established ATN on duration of renal failure, requirement for dialysis, or survival (11). The increase in urine output in this setting is caused by decreased tubular reabsorption in residual functioning nephrons (not recruitment of nonfunctioning nephrons), volume expansion (initial sodium retention), and urea osmotic diuresis.

A number of studies have suggested worsened outcomes in ATN with the use of loop diuretics in the setting of contrast media (9, 12) and cardiac surgery. A systematic review (13, 14) comparing fluids alone with diuretics found no evidence of improvement in survival, incidence of ARF, or need for renal replacement therapy (RRT). Deafness, possibly permanent, is a known complication of high-dose loop diuretics.

Mannitol

Mannitol may preserve mitochondrial function by minimizing postinjury edema. Human trials have failed to show benefit in reducing ARF with mannitol versus fluid alone in rhabdomyolysis (15), cardiac surgery (16), and vascular and biliary tract surgery (17). A trend toward harm was noted in the prevention of contrast nephropathy (12).

Dopamine Agonists

Dopamine has a number of effects in the kidney via dopamine A1 and A2 receptors. In the proximal tubule, dopamine, via the generation of cyclic AMP, decreases Na^+-H^+ exchange and the Na^+-H^+-ATPase pump, thus, decreasing sodium reabsorption. In the collecting tubules, this effect on Na^+-H^+-ATPase and decreased aldosterone secretion reduces sodium reabsorption (18).

When infused in doses of 0.5 to 3 µg/kg/min, dopamine causes afferent and efferent glomerular arteriolar dilatation, increasing blood flow with little or no increase in GFR. At higher concentrations, dopamine causes vasoconstriction via α-adrenergic receptors.

There is no evidence in human studies for a "renal protective effect" of dopamine.

- In 1994, Baldwin et al. studied the effect of postoperative low-dose dopamine on renal function after major elective vascular surgery. Patients were administered saline or saline plus dopamine as fluid replacement. No difference in renal function was demonstrated between the two groups (19).
- In the North American Study of the Safety and Efficacy of Murine Monoclonal Antibody to Tumor Necrosis Factor for the Treatment of Septic Shock (NORASEPT) II study, 400 patients with septic shock and oliguria nonrandomly received no, low-, or high-dose dopamine.

The incidence of ARF and requirement for RRT was not significant different between groups (20).
- A large randomized controlled trial of low-dose dopamine in 328 critically ill patients with impaired creatinine, oliguria, and at least two systemic inflammatory response syndrome (SIRS) criteria failed to show any benefit in progression, need for RRT, or death (21).
- Studies of fenoldopam, a relatively selective dopamine A1 receptor agonist, although shown to increase sodium excretion and renal blood flow in healthy and hypertensive patients, has not shown benefit in ARF in the critically ill (22).

N-Acetylcysteine

N-Acetylcysteine (NAC) has been shown in a number of studies to decrease the incidence of contrast nephropathy in high-risk patients (23, 24), but without improvement in RRT requirement or survival. Importantly, NAC may decrease creatinine via activation of creatinine kinase (25) but not GFR. Promising studies have led to the introduction of protocols in many institutions for the prophylactic use of NAC in the prevention of contrast-induced nephropathy. With few side effects, low cost, and ease of administration (oral or intravenous), many centers have erred on the side of possible benefit in the face of lack of hard evidence of long-term benefit (26).

Others

Trials have failed to demonstrate benefit of *natriuretic peptides* (10, 27) or *adenosine agonists* (28). Experimental therapies, such as antioxidants and erythropoietin are unproven in humans.

In the absence of further evidence, fluids, and possibly NAC, are the gold standards of interventional strategies.

Supportive Strategies

Fluid resuscitation and correction of hypotension are clearly essential. There is no evidence of advantage of one particular *inotrope* over another.

No evidence exists that reversing hypotension with noradrenaline compromises mesenteric or renal blood flow (29).

Van den Berghe demonstrated that tight *glucose control* with intravenous therapy improved outcomes in critically ill patients, including decreased incidence of ARF (30, 31).

Nutritional support of the critically ill is the basic standard of care, although not always achieved. Early enteral nutrition is supported by meta-analyses of Level II trials; benefits include preservation of muscle mass, the maintenance of the gastrointestinal mucosal barrier and immune status, and a possible reduction in multiorgan dysfunction (32–34). A Level I trial is currently planned by the Australian and New Zealand Intensive Care Society (ANZICS) clinical trials group comparing early enteral nutrition with standard care in 1470 critically ill patients intolerant of early enteral nutrition (www.actr.org.au).

There is no evidence to support *prophylactic hemofiltration* to prevent contrast nephropathy, despite filtration removal of contrast.

Early recognition and adequate management of the deteriorating clinical condition of a patient is fundamental in the prevention of morbidity and mortality, including ARF. In a hospital-based study of a medical emergency team (MET) system, Bellomo et al. demonstrated reduced incidence of postoperative adverse outcomes, mortality rate, and mean hospital length of stay (35). This was not validated in a larger cluster-randomized controlled trial of 23 hospitals with no effect on incidence of cardiac arrest, unplanned admissions to ICU, or unexpected death (36). Nevertheless, the principles of early recognition, monitoring, and adequate response remain fundamental.

Postinjury Prevention of ARF

Secondary renal injury occurs after the primary insult has triggered the initial injury to the kidneys.

Strategies for postinjury prevention of ARF overlap with those of primary prevention (37) as described above. They include maintenance of adequate intravascular volume, cardiac output, mean arterial blood pressure (MAP), avoidance of further insult, and supportive strategies.

Assessment and Correction of Volume Depletion

Clinical signs of relative or absolute volume depletion include loss of tissue turgor, hypotension, postural hypotension, and decreased venous pressure (reduced jugular venous pressure). Although left ventricular end diastolic pressure (LVEDP) is the most important determinant of left ventricular output and, thus, tissue perfusion, central venous pressure is useful because it has a direct relationship to LVEDP, with the exceptions of pure left-sided or pure right-sided failure (cor pulmonale). Other clinical manifestations may be specific to the source of depletion (losses or third space sequestration), type of fluid lost, and to the associated electrolyte and acid-base abnormalities.

Recently, Vincent proposed a protocol for routine fluid challenge with defined rules based on clinical response to the volumes infused, allowing for prompt deficit correction while minimizing risks of fluid overload (38).

Maintenance of Adequate MAP and Cardiac Output

There is currently insufficient data to recommend firm therapeutic targets, suffice to say, Level III evidence suggests failure to maintain systolic blood pressure greater than 80 mmHg or MAP greater than 50 mmHg is associated with increased risk of developing ARF (39). A low cardiac output is a major risk factor for ARF after cardiac surgery (40), but supranormal cardiac output has no beneficial effect.

Avoidance of Further Insults

Appropriate dosage of medication and avoidance (or protective strategies) of nephrotoxins is advised.

Renal Replacement Therapy

Intermittent versus continuous renal replacement strategies and dose delivery are discussed in a later chapter.

TABLE 5.2. Summary of guidelines for management of ARF

Make diagnosis	
Exclusion of prerenal causes	E.g., volume depletion, cardiac and liver disease, nephrotoxins
Exclusion of postrenal causes	Renal ultrasound
Exclusion of intrinsic renal causes	E.g., review urinary sediment, consider renal biopsy
Evaluation of urinary electrolytes	Only in the absence of diuretics
Treat reversible causes	
Volume resuscitation	Maintain fluid balance but avoid overload
Blood pressure support	Inotropic if necessary, however no validated physiological targets or end points have been established
Treat electrolyte complications	E.g., hyperkalemia
No dopamine	
Address/avoid exacerbating factors	
Treatment of underlying etiology	E.g., treat sepsis, further investigation if diagnosis unclear, surgical referral if appropriate
Adjust medication dosage	Discontinue any nephrotoxic drugs
Avoid further renal insult	E.g., minimize contrast-induced injury with fluids and consider NAC
Optimize "kidney's environment"	
Maintain renal perfusion	Maintain fluid balance, blood pressure, and cardiac output
Adequate nutrition	
Glucose control	
Appropriate RRT	Timely introduction of RRT, avoidance of complications (e.g., hypotension, line-related sepsis, biocompatible dialysis membranes), and appropriate dose of dialysis
Other	
Constantly review diagnosis, which may multifactorial in nature	Consider further investigations, e.g., renal biopsy and radiological investigations, as appropriate
Appropriate medical review	E.g., MET resources, nephrology input

Summary

Measures of severity of illness are limited when applied to patients with ARF and, at present, none are currently adequate to predict mortality of ARF (41). In the light of available evidence, guidelines for the management of ARF have been formulated and given in Table 5.2. Admiral efforts to clearly define levels of injury in ARF and physiological end points (42) will enable further research into prevention, amelioration, and management of ARF and, thus, impact on the significant associated morbidity and mortality.

References

1. Levy EM, Viscoli CM, Horwitz RI. The effect of acute renal failure on mortality. A cohort analysis. *JAMA.* 1996; 275(19): 1489–1494.
2. Kellum JA. Acute renal failure, interdisciplinary knowledge and the need for standardization. *Curr Opin Crit Care.* 2005; 11(6): 525–526.
3. Liano G, Pascual J. Acute renal failure. Madrid Acute Renal Failure Study Group. *Lancet.* 1996; 347(8999): 479.
4. Herget-Rosenthal S, Marggraf G, Husing J, et al. Early detection of acute renal failure by serum cystatin C. *Kidney Int.* 2004; 66(3): 1115–1122.
5. Madaio MP. Renal biopsy. *Kidney Int.* 1990; 38(3): 529–543.
6. Mueller C, Buerkle G, Buettner HJ, et al. Prevention of contrast media-associated nephropathy: randomized comparison of 2 hydration regimens in 1620 patients undergoing coronary angioplasty. *Arch Intern Med.* 2002; 162(3): 329–336.
7. Kellum JA, Leblanc M, Gibney RT, et al. Primary prevention of acute renal failure in the critically ill. *Curr Opin Crit Care.* 2005; 11(6): 537–541.
8. Rahman SN, Conger JD. Glomerular and tubular factors in urine flow rates of acute renal failure patients. *Am J Kidney Dis.* 1994; 23(6): 788–793.
9. Lassnigg A, Donner E, Grubhofer G, et al. Lack of renoprotective effects of dopamine and furosemide during cardiac surgery. *J Am Soc Nephrol.* 2000; 11(1): 97–104.

TABLE 6.3. Specific tests to consider in determining the cause of ARF in surgical patients[a]

Blood tests	Creatinine kinase	To exclude rhabdomyolysis especially after trauma
	Full blood count	Eosinophilia is seen in 80% of patients with drug-induced interstitial nephritis
Urinalysis	Dipstick	Significant proteinuria/hematuria/casts suggest intrinsic renal pathology
	Biochemistry	Urinary sodium and osmolality to help differentiate prerenal failure from ATN
	Culture	To exclude urinary tract infection
Diagnostic imaging	Ultrasound scan	To exclude obstruction and to determine renal size
	Imaging of renal perfusion (e.g., renal Dopplers, computed tomographic angiogram, MAG3, DTPA)	Renal vascular supply may be of concern after major abdominal aortic surgery. Investigation will depend on patient stability and local resources
Measurement of intravesical pressure		To exclude intra-abdominal hypertension and compartment syndrome

[a]MAG3, mercaptoacetyltriglycine; DTPA, diethylene triamine pentaacetic acid.

failure is still conflicting. Although low cardiac output has been shown to be a strong risk factor for ARF after cardiac surgery, there is no evidence that increasing cardiac output from adequate to supranormal has beneficial renal effects.

Vascular Surgery

Patients undergoing vascular surgery generally represent a high-risk group for renal failure. The exact incidence of renal injury in this context is unknown but, again, depends on the definition of renal injury, patient characteristics, and type of surgery. Open surgical repair of abdominal aneurysms is associated with a high risk of renal failure, especially with suprarenal aortic cross clamping, massive bleeding, or cholesterol embolization. The emergence of endovascular repair has led to a reduced incidence of ARF, however, the risk is not completely abolished by vascular stents. In rare instances, endovascular stents have been found to migrate, resulting in occlusion of arterial orifices, including renal arteries.

Urological Surgery

Obstruction is a common cause of ARF in patients with urological problems. Although this diagnosis is usually made before surgery, it may occur postoperatively (e.g., after renal transplantation or ureteric surgery). In general, the majority of ARF posturological surgery is because of acute tubular necrosis precipitated by hypotension,

volume depletion, bleeding complications, and/or urosepsis.

Diagnosis (Table 6.3)

At present, there are no universally accepted criteria for the definition of ARF. Most arbitrary definitions are based on a rise in serum creatinine or fall in calculated creatinine clearance. It is important to remember that the glomerular filtration rate has to fall to less than 50% before serum creatinine rises, which means that any rise in serum creatinine always implies significant renal injury.

Treatment

General Measures

• Restoration of renal perfusion pressure
• Correction of volume depletion
• Avoidance of hypotension (including *relative* hypotension). Be guided by the patient's preexisting blood pressure
• Fluid resuscitation, as appropriate, and use of vasopressor agents if perfusing pressure still inadequate
• Optimal treatment of sepsis/septic shock
• Avoidance of nephrotoxic medication if possible. Close monitoring of drug levels when aminoglycosides are necessary

- Renal replacement therapy in case of severe metabolic acidosis, unresponsive fluid overload, resistant hyperkalemia, or pericarditis
- Early involvement of nephrologists if an intrinsic cause of renal failure is a possibility or if the patient is likely to require ongoing renal support

Specific Measures

- Removal of septic focus if possible (e.g. drainage of intra-abdominal abscess)
- Relief of obstruction
- Management of abdominal compartment syndrome (including consideration of abdominal decompression)
- Revascularization of kidneys, if appropriate

Treatments that Have Not Been Shown to Alter the Course of ARF

- Diuretics (unless patient is fluid overloaded)
- Low-dose dopamine

Vasopressor Agents and the Kidney

Vasopressor agents are often needed to manage septic shock, and noradrenaline and dopamine are good first-line drugs. Although there are few direct comparison studies, patients with septic shock tend to respond better to noradrenaline. Concern regarding the potential for noradrenaline to impair renal and mesenteric perfusion has been reduced by studies showing that reversal of hypotension with noradrenaline outweighed this effect and increased renal and mesenteric perfusion.

Prevention

General Vigilance

Meticulous attention to fluid balance, blood pressure, prescribed drugs, and treatment of sepsis are the most important preventive measures. There is insufficient evidence to recommend specific physiological targets (MAP, cardiac output, filling pressures) that will ensure adequate renal perfusion. Instead, therapy needs to be individualized based on the baseline physiological condition of the individual patient.

Early Resuscitation

Early recognition of patients at risk and timely resuscitation has been shown to result in significant reduction of the development of ARF.

Prevention of Contrast-Induced Nephropathy

The administration of fluids has been shown to be the most important factor in prevention of contrast-induced renal injury. Although the optimal fluid regimen is uncertain, available data support a regimen of 0.9% saline at 1 mL/kg/h intravenously from up to 12 hours before administration of contrast medium and for up to 12 hours after. Studies on the prophylactic role of N-acetylcysteine have had conflicting results. Meta-analyses have concluded that prophylactic N-acetylcysteine was harmless and may prevent an acute rise of serum creatinine after intravenous contrast, but survival and need for dialysis were not affected.

Tight Glucose Control

A single-center randomized controlled trial on intensive insulin therapy in postoperative ventilated patients showed a 41% decrease in the incidence of ARF requiring dialysis in the group of patients whose blood sugars were tightly controlled between 4.4 and 6.1 mmol/L compared with patients whose blood sugar was allowed to rise to 12 mmol/L before insulin was initiated. Further studies are necessary to confirm these results.

Prophylactic Dopamine or Diuretics

A recent meta-analysis of 61 trials showed that low-dose dopamine (<5 μg/kg/min) often increased urine output but had no effect on renal function or prevention of ARF.

Natriuretic Peptides

Urodilatin (renal natriuretic peptide) or anaritide (synthetic form of atrial natriuretic peptide) have failed to show any protective effect on the kidney.

Future Advances

At present, no agents have conclusively demonstrated a protective effect against ARF or alteration of the course of ARF. Strategies aimed at modulating renal function and renal recovery have focused on several mechanisms:

1. Reduction of renal metabolism and energy consumption of the kidneys (i.e., induction of hypothermia, use of insulin-like factor I).
2. Modulation of the inflammatory system (i.e., up-regulation of the acute stress response, manipulation of complement system, blockade of adhesion molecules).
3. Ischemic preconditioning.

These strategies are clearly important areas of research but not ready for clinical application.

References

1. Bahar I, Akgul A, Ozatik MA, Vural KM, Demirbag AE, Boran M, Tasdemir O. Acute renal failure following open heart surgery: risk factors and prognosis. *Perfusion* 2005; 20: 317–322.
2. Barrett BJ, Parfrey PS. Preventing nephropathy induced by contrast medium. *N Engl J Med* 2006; 354: 379–386.
3. Chertow GM, Levy EM, Hammermeister KE, Grover F, Daley J. Independent association between acute renal failure and mortality following cardiac surgery. *Am J Med* 1998; 104: 343–348.
4. Friedrich JO, Adhikari N, Herridge MS, Beyene J. Meta-analysis: low-dose dopamine increases urine output but does not prevent renal dysfunction or death. *Ann Intern Med* 2005; 142: 510–524.
5. Lassnigg A, Donner E, Grubhofer G, Presterl E, Druml W, Hiesmayr M. Lack of renoprotective effects of dopamine and furosemide during cardiac surgery. *J Am Soc Nephrol* 2000; 11: 97–104.
6. Mangano DT, Tudor IC, Dietzel C. Multicenter Study of Perioperative Ischemia Research Group; Ischemia Research and Education Foundation. The risk associated with aprotinin in cardiac surgery. *N Engl J Med* 2006; 354: 353–365.
7. Van den Berghe G, Wouters PJ, Bouillon R, et al. Intensive insulin therapy in critically ill patients. *N Engl J Med* 2001; 345: 1359–1367.

7
Rhabdomyolysis and Compartment Syndrome

Laurie Tomlinson and Stephen Holt

Rhabdomyolysis occurs when an insult causing myocyte necrosis results in release of intracellular contents into the circulation. Renal dysfunction is caused by a combination of renal vasoconstriction, tubular damage, and tubular obstruction.

Causes

Rhabdomyolysis accounts for approximately 7% of all causes of acute renal failure (ARF) during peacetime. This figure is much higher after natural disasters and in wartime. For example, after the 1998 Turkish earthquake, 12% of the hospitalized population developed significant renal dysfunction and 477 patients required dialysis.

Direct crush or compression injury and drugs are the most important causes in clinical practice, see Table 7.1. There are often predisposing factors, for example, alcohol, which can presensitize myocytes so they may be damaged by a more trivial insult. A clinical scoring system exists (not widely used) based on levels of phosphate, potassium, albumin, creatine kinase (CK), and presence of dehydration and sepsis.

Compartment Syndrome

After an appropriate precipitant, inflammation within a muscular compartment causes a vicious cycle of increasing pressure. This leads to further inflammation and damage, eventually compromising blood supply, leading to further muscle necrosis. There may be severe pain, with loss of muscle function and loss of distal pulses. The diagnosis may be occult, especially in the unconscious patient. Direct pressure measurements can be made by passing a needle connected to a pressure manometer (e.g., central venous pressure [CVP] transducer) into the affected muscle compartment.

A fasciotomy should be considered if the pressure exceeds 40 mmHg or greater than 30 mmHg above diastolic pressure.

Diagnosis

Serum changes consequent on rhabdomyolysis:

Creatine Kinase

Very high levels of the muscle enzyme CK are pathognomic of this condition. The degree of elevation is proportional to the degree of muscle injury. Other muscle enzymes, such as aspartate transaminase (AST) and lactate dehydrogenase (LDH) are also elevated. CK levels should decline by approximately 40% per day, a plateau or an increase should prompt a search for ongoing muscle damage.

Hyperkalemia

Hyperkalemia caused by efflux of potassium from damaged cells is an early and life-threatening consequence of rhabdomyolysis. It should be aggressively treated.

TABLE 7.1. Causes of rhabdomyolysis

Physical	**Trauma**, hyperthermia, hypothermia, exercise, electric shock, seizures, delirium tremens
Toxins and drugs	**Alcohol**, **statins**, amphetamines, aspirin (overdose), barium, barbiturates, caffeine, carbon monoxide, ecstasy, ethylene glycol, LSD, malignant hyperpyrexia, neuroleptic malignant syndrome, opiates, toluene, snake/insect bites, vasopressin
Muscle ischemia	Vascular ischemia, coma, sickle cell disease, surgery, vasoconstrictors, CO_2 angiography
Infection	Virtually any viral or bacterial infection (e.g., influenza, HIV, Epstein-Barr virus, *Legionella*, tetanus, malaria, *Bacillus cereus*)
Metabolic	Hypernatremia/**hyponatremia**, hypokalemia, hypophosphatemia, diabetic ketoacidosis, diabetic hyperosmolar coma, water intoxication, myxedema
Inherited	Deficiency of carnitine palmityl transferase II, phosphofructokinase, myophosphorylase (McArdles), myoadenylate deaminase, cytochrome oxidase, succinic dehydrogenase, coenzyme Q10 deficiency, King-Denborough Syndrome, Wilson's disease
Immune	Polymyositis, dermatomyositis

Acidosis

Metabolic acidosis may be caused by increased lactate production and lactate release by damaged muscle. Myoglobin (Mb) is considerably more toxic in an acid milieu.

Early Hypocalcemia and Late Hypercalcemia

Serum calcium levels often fall dramatically, with total calcium less than 1.7 mmol/L in the early stages. This is caused by sequestration into damaged muscle and reperfusion-induced cellular calcium uptake. In contrast, intracellular calcium concentrations in damaged muscle may rise by up to 10-fold. In the recovery phase of rhabdomyolysis, serum calcium levels normalize and may even "overshoot," secondary to calcium release by recovering myocytes and a transient rise in parathyroid hormone (a reflex to the initial hypocalcemia).

*Symptoms of **hypocalcemia** are rare and treatment with intravenous calcium should be avoided unless tetany or cardiac dysfunction is present. Pharmacologically administered calcium is taken up avidly by the damaged muscle. It may be deposited as inorganic complexes causing "heterotopic calcification," which delays recovery and can lead to long-term muscle dysfunction.*

Hyperphosphatemia

Serum phosphate often exceeds 3 mmol/L.

Urinary Abnormalities

Urine dipsticks are usually positive for blood because they detect the heme moiety present in both hemoglobin (Hb) and Mb. On microscopy, few red cells are seen (unless there is coexistent trauma), instead, the characteristic "brown sugar casts" of Mb are seen (Figure 7.1). When there is uncertainty, Mb can be specifically assayed in the urine, although it has a short half-life. An assay exists for myosin heavy chain, which remains positive for up to 12 days after the initial insult.

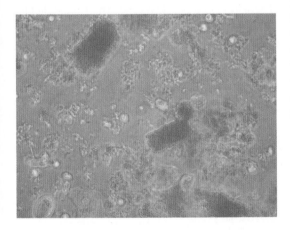

FIGURE 7.1. "Brown sugar" Mb casts under light microscope are similar to granular casts but have a brown/rusty tinge. Additional red cells, tubular cells, and other debris are also present within the urine.

Pathophysiology of ARF

Suggested causes:

1. **A reduction in renal blood flow.** There is a reduction in the effective blood volume caused by fluid shifts from the intravascular to extracellular fluid compartments. Mb binds to nitric oxide (NO), preventing intrarenal vasodilation

(especially in the medulla) and, in addition, vaso-dilators (e.g., endothelin) are increased.

2. **Direct heme protein tubulotoxicity** occurs, probably by free radical-mediated mechanisms.

3. **Tubular cast formation.** Urinary Mb and Tamm-Horsfall protein (THP) complex and precipitate as tubular casts. These casts are less soluble in acidic conditions. Although there is some evidence that these complexes cause tubular obstruction, micropuncture studies have shown relatively low intratubular pressures, suggesting that these casts are as a result of reduced tubular flow and reduced washout rather than by obstruction per se.

Treatment

Intravascular Volume Expansion

Intravascular volume expansion at the first possible opportunity after the insult is the single most effective therapeutic maneuver in rhabdomyolysis. This not only prevents or limits renal damage but may play a role in preventing acidosis and limiting ongoing damage caused by hypoperfusion. Very large volumes of fluid can be lost into areas of muscle injury. In trauma situations in which there is a risk of crush injury, fluid resuscitation should be commenced before the victim is extricated.

Alkalinization

There is much compelling evidence to suggest that urinary alkalinization greatly reduces the nephrotoxicity of Mb. However, there are no large human trials that confirm this consistent finding from animal research. The potential benefits in this setting include reduced renal vasoconstriction, a dramatic reduction in the ability of Mb to cause oxidant damage, and increased solubility of Mb-THP complex.

Alkalinization can lower ionized calcium still further and, if administered, it is wise to periodically check the ionized calcium.

A suggested fluid replacement regime would be:

- Isotonic bicarbonate (1.26% sodium bicarbonate) until urine pH is greater than 7 if the patient is intravascularly volume deplete (which is usual)

- Bicarbonate solutions that are more concentrated can be administered in small aliquots, e.g., 50 mL of 8.4% $NaHCO_3$ via central access in patients who are intravascularly full—remembering that this is 1 mmol of sodium per milliliter of fluid and may cause sodium/fluid overload

Mannitol

Mannitol promotes an osmotic diuresis and may reduce pressure in a swollen muscle compartment, but it also causes osmotically induced tubular damage with vacuolation. There is no good evidence that it is more effective than saline alone and it has little scientific rationale to recommend its routine use.

Dialysis/Hemofiltration

The circulating concentration of Mb can be reduced by hemofiltration, plasma exchange, and hemodialysis, with dialysis being somewhat less successful. It has not been shown that any physical therapy materially reduces renal Mb burden or shortens the duration of renal replacement therapy. Physical therapies may have a role, if commenced early, or if Mb release can be anticipated, such as during arterial surgery.

Prognosis

There is an unquantifiable early mortality, mainly caused by hyperkalemia or the insult. Mortality after diagnosis is up to 20%, usually caused by other associated conditions, e.g., sepsis. Survivors of the Japanese earthquake in 1995 arriving in hospital within 6 hours had an approximately 20% chance of developing ARF, whereas all of those arriving after 40 hours developed renal failure. If the patient recovers from the initial insult, the renal dysfunction almost always resolves, but can take up to 3 months.

Summary

- Rhabdomyolysis is a common cause of ARF, with important early biochemical changes that may be fatal if treatment is not instituted quickly

9
Therapeutic Plasma Exchange

Tim Leach

Therapeutic plasma exchange (TPE) is an extra-corporeal blood purification technique designed for the removal of large molecular weight substances from plasma. Large molecular weight substances equilibrate slowly between the vascular space and the interstitium. Calculations of the rate of their removal by TPE follows first-order kinetics, i.e., approximately 60% is removed by a single plasma volume exchange, and 75% by an exchange equal to 1.4 times the plasma volume.

Blood is pumped through a highly permeable filter, replacing the filtrate with fluid as indicated (Table 9.1). Venous access on the intensive care unit (ICU) is via a double-lumen dialysis catheter, but can be via two wide-gauge peripheral venous cannulae. If chronic therapy is indicated, an arteriovenous fistula is used. The patient and filter are anticoagulated during the procedure.

Indications (Table 9.2)

The basic premise of TPE is that removal of large molecular weight substances from the circulation will reduce further damage and may permit reversal of the pathological process.

Other benefits include unloading the reticuloendothelial system to permit further endogenous removal of circulating toxins, stimulation of lymphocyte clones, and allowing re-infusion of large volumes of plasma without the risk of volume overload.

For TPE to be appropriate, the substance to be removed should be:

- Of molecular weight greater than 15,000 kDa so it cannot be removed in any other way, and/or
- Of sufficient half-life that TPE is quicker than endogenous removal, and/or
- Acutely toxic and resistant to conventional therapy

Prescription (Table 9.1)

Calculation of plasma volume:

$$\text{Estimated plasma volume (L)} = 0.07 \times \text{Weight (kg)} \times (1 - \text{hematocrit})$$

1. Before each treatment, measure serum potassium calcium and clotting screen.
2. Calculate the estimated plasma volume: Volume of exchange is measured in Patient Plasma Volumes (~3 L).
3. Prescribe the plasma exchange:
   a. Number and spacing of treatments
   b. Volume and type of fluid
4. Electrolyte supplementation as needed (potassium and calcium).
5. If coagulopathic consider, fresh-frozen plasma (FFP) as the final exchange volume.

After Procedure

- Repeat electrolytes and clotting after 2 hours and increase supplementation as needed
- FFP can be given as the final exchange volume if coagulopathic

TABLE 9.1. Example of TPE prescription[a]

Indication	Plasma volumes	Replacement fluid	Number of exchanges	Exchange frequency
Rapidly progressive glomerulonephritis Acute renal failure caused by myeloma kidney	1 to 1.5	Albumin, with FFP if pulmonary hemorrhage	7 to 10	Daily or alternate days
Hyperviscosity Syndrome	1	Albumin/saline mixture[b]	Until symptoms subside or plasma viscosity normal	Daily
Anti-glomerular basement membrane (GBM) disease	1.5	Albumin, with FFP if pulmonary hemorrhage	7 to 10	Daily
Hemolytic uremic syndrome/thrombotic thrombocytopenic purpura	1 to 2	All FFP	Until platelets normal/no red cell fragments (usually 7 to 16)	Once or twice daily
Guillain-Barré Syndrome	2	Albumin	4	Alternate days

[a]From: Wessex Renal and Transplant Unit, United Kingdom.
[b]No more than one part saline to two parts albumin (i.e., ≤1 L saline for 2 L albumin).

TABLE 9.2. American Association of Blood Banks indications for TPE

1. *Standard and acceptable*
   - Chronic inflammatory demyelinating polyneuropathy
   - Cryoglobulinemia
   - Anti-GBM disease
   - Guillain-Barré syndrome
   - Familial hypercholesterolemia
   - Myasthenia gravis
   - Posttransfusion purpura
   - Thrombotic thrombocytopenic purpura

2. *Sufficient evidence to suggest efficacy/acceptable adjunct*
   - Cold agglutinin disease
   - Protein-bound toxins (drug overdose/ poisonings)
   - Hemolytic uremic syndrome
   - Rapidly progressive glomerulonephritis
   - Systemic vasculitis
   - Acute renal failure caused by myeloma kidney

3. *Inconclusive evidence or uncertain benefit-to-risk ratio*
   - ABO-incompatible organ or marrow transplantation
   - Coagulation factor inhibitors
   - Idiopathic thrombocytopenic purpura
   - Multiple sclerosis
   - Progressive systemic sclerosis
   - Thyroid storm
   - Warm autoimmune hemolytic anemia

4. ***No*** *efficacy in trials*
   - AIDS
   - Amyotrophic lateral sclerosis
   - Dermato/polymyositis
   - Psoriasis
   - Renal transplant rejection
   - Rheumatoid arthritis
   - Schizophrenia

Complications

- Hypotension: vasovagal, hypovolemia
- Fluid overload
- Hypocalcemia causing tetany
- Hypokalemia
- Coagulopathy caused by removal of clotting factors or thrombocytopenia with heparin anticoagulation
- Protein-bound drug removal (administer drugs *after* TPE)
- ACE inhibitors may cause flushing and hypotension (stop 24 h before treatment)

10
Renal Replacement Therapy

John H. Reeves

Acute renal failure (ARF) occurs in 7% of patients admitted to the intensive care unit (ICU) (1). Previously, mortality exceeded 91%, but with the introduction of dialysis, this quickly fell to approximately 50% (2). Overall mortality for ARF has remained approximately 50%, associated with increasing comorbidity (3).

There is no specific therapy for ARF other than removal of the cause and ongoing supportive care awaiting spontaneous recovery. Renal replacement therapy (RRT) is the cornerstone of that supportive care.

The Basics

Extracorporeal RRT involves the passage of a patient's blood outside his/her body through a dialysis or hemofilter machine, where the removal of unwanted solutes and excess water and the replacement of lost bicarbonate (or buffer base) take place. The "purified" blood is returned to the patient.

Clearance can be defined as that volume of plasma completely cleared of a substance in a given time. During extracorporeal RRT, net solute clearance can be achieved by ultrafiltration across a porous membrane down a pressure gradient (*filtration*), or by diffusion across a semipermeable membrane down a concentration gradient (*dialysis*), or both. During filtration, the filtrate is discarded and a replacement solution is added to the blood to maintain fluid and electrolyte equilibrium. During dialysis, a continuous stream of dialysate is passed in the opposite direction to blood, on the nonblood side of the membrane, to maintain a concentration gradient favoring the out-diffusion of unwanted solutes. Both dialysate and replacement solutions contain electrolytes in physiological concentrations and some form of buffer base.

The *hemofilter* or dialysis membrane's permeability to water is determined by its surface area (typically 0.5 to 2.0 m²) and the number and size of its pores (typically 0.0055-μm diameter in a high-flux hemofilter). The pore size determines the size of molecules that are freely filtered along with water. Current hemofilters freely filter substances up to approximately 5000-D molecular weight and then in decreasing amounts up to a cut off of approximately 20,000 Da. This minimizes loss of important larger molecules, such as albumin (molecular weight, 57,000 Da).

The ratio between the concentration of solute in filtrate and that in plasma water is called the *sieving coefficient*, and this concept becomes important in calculating the clearance of intermediate-sized molecules. The sieving coefficient for a small unbound solutes is one, decreasing to zero as molecular size and or plasma protein binding increases.

Theoretical small solute clearance can be predicted by knowledge of the blood flow through the extracorporeal circuit (Q_B) and the rate of ultrafiltration (Q_F) and dialysate flow (Q_D) (Figure 10.1).

During *continuous* RRT (CRRT), when blood flow is significantly higher than dialysate or ultrafiltration rates, small solute clearance is determined by dialysate and ultrafiltrate flow. Assuming complete concentration equilibrium between dialysate and plasma water and a sieving coefficient equal to one:

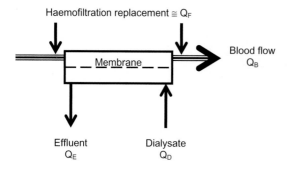

Haemofiltration replacement $\cong Q_F$

Membrane

Blood flow Q_B

Effluent Q_E

Dialysate Q_D

Figure 10.1. Predicting clearance during RRT.

week. In contrast, ICU patients with ARF may require daily treatment (7).

Hybrid: there is increasing interest in hybrid approaches for extracorporeal RRT in the ICU (8, 9). For example, during sustained low-efficiency dialysis (SLED), daily intermittent therapy is reduced in intensity and extended in duration up to 8 or 12 hours. The regular breaks aid staffing and free patients for investigations and procedures. The reduced intensity reduces the cardiorespiratory destabilization associated with IHD.

$$\text{Clearance during CRRT} = QF + QD = QE$$

In contrast, during *intermittent* hemodialysis (IHD), dialysate flow is significantly higher than blood flow, and blood flow becomes the limiting factor for solute clearance. Small solute clearance is proportional to the plasma flow through the dialyzer:

$$\text{Clearance during IHD} \cong QB \times (1 - \text{hematocrit})$$

This simplified analysis only holds for small, unbound solutes, such as urea and creatinine. Increasing molecular weight decreases diffusive clearance more significantly than convective clearance. Binding to macromolecules, such as albumin, decreases convective and diffusive clearance (4).

Classification of RRT

In 1977, when Peter Kramer first described continuous arteriovenous hemofiltration (CAVH) as a therapy for diuretic resistant fluid overload (5), the only other types of RRT were IHD and peritoneal dialysis (PD). Since then, the classification of RRT has expanded (6). See the glossary in Table 10.1.

Duration or Timing of Therapy

Continuous: CRRT aims to provide support 24 h/d, but, in practice, is interrupted by factors such as patient transfer out of the ICU or circuit failure.

Intermittent: IHD requires approximately 3 hours per treatment. Patients with end-stage renal failure (ESRF) may be maintained in the community with as few as three dialysis sessions per

Access

Arteriovenous: arteriovenous access involves cannulation of a medium-sized artery and large vein—often the femoral artery and vein. Blood flows passively from the artery through the extracorporeal circuit (ECC) and back through the vein, driven by the mean arterial pressure. This method is reserved for situations in which resources are limited.

Venovenous: venovenous access involves cannulation of central veins, most commonly with a double-lumen cannula in the femoral, internal jugular, or subclavian vein. Blood flow is driven by a pump in the ECC. This increases reliability of blood flow and maximizes solute clearance, but introduces the need for more complex safety mechanisms to detect fault conditions, such as air embolism or circuit occlusion.

Mechanism of Solute Removal

Convection: when solute is cleared by ultrafiltration through a porous membrane, we say that the clearance of the solute is *convective*—carried by the bulk flow of plasma water. During CRRT, the process is called *hemofiltration*.

Diffusion: when solute is cleared by diffusion down a concentration gradient across a semipermeable membrane, we say that the clearance of the solute is *diffusive*. The process is called *hemodialysis*.

Combinations: diafiltration is the term applied when both convection and diffusion are operating to remove solute.

Adsorption: adsorption is the binding of substances to the membrane under molecular

TABLE 10.1. RRT: A glossary[a]

Acronym	Full Name	Notes	Seed reference
SCUF	Slow continuous ultrafiltration	AV or VV	Silverstein 1974 (12)
CAVH	Continuous arteriovenous hemofiltration		Kramer 1977 (5)
CAVHD	Continuous arteriovenous hemodialysis		
CAVHDF	Continuous arteriovenous hemodiafiltration		
CVVH	Continuous venovenous hemofiltration		
CVVHD	Continuous venovenous hemodialysis		
CVVHDF	Continuous venovenous hemodiafiltration		
CHFD	Continuous high flux dialysis	AV or VV	Ronco 1996 (13)
HVHF	High volume hemofiltration	AV or VV	Cole 2001 (14)
CPF	Continuous plasma filtration	AV or VV	Reeves 1999 (15)
CPFA	Coupled plasma filtration adsorption	AV or VV	Ronco 2003 (16)
SLED	Sustained low efficiency dialysis		Marshall 2004 (17)
EDD	Extended daily dialysis		Kumar 2000 (18)
PDIRRT	Prolonged daily intermittent RRT		Naka 2004 (9)

[a]AV, arteriovenous; VV, venovenous.

attraction. Adsorption is used specifically for toxin removal using activated charcoal cartridges (10) and it is being tested as a means of blood purification in sepsis (11).

Intensity of Therapy

For example, slow continuous ultrafiltration (SCUF) is performed to simply remove excess extracellular fluid. High-volume hemofiltration (HVHF) is used to intentionally accelerate the clearance of target mediators, and high-flux dialysis (HFD) (dialysis performed with highly permeable membranes) is designed to accelerate the clearance of urea and larger molecules.

Indications for RRT

"Traditional" indications (19)

- Diuretic resistant fluid overload
- Life-threatening hyperkalemia
- Severe metabolic acidosis
- Symptomatic uremia

Kramer's original description of CAVH involved the treatment of diuretic resistant fluid overload (5). During the intervening years, there has been controversy surrounding the use of diuretics in ARF (20), but they may be helpful in the fluid management of ARF before the institution of RRT (21, 22).

There is little information regarding what specific threshold plasma concentrations of potassium, bicarbonate, urea, or creatinine should be used for the institution of RRT. In a retrospective comparison of early versus late CRRT in trauma associated ARF, Gettings et al. (23) found that patients in whom CRRT was commenced at a mean blood urea nitrogen (BUN) of 42.6 mg/dL (15.2 mmol/L) had a survival rate of 39% compared with 20% in patients in whom the mean BUN at commencement was 94.5 mg/dL (33.7 mmol/L).

"Nonrenal" Indications

- Drug and toxin removal
- Sepsis and septic shock
- Inborn errors of metabolism
- Congestive cardiac failure
- Cerebral edema

IHD can accelerate the elimination of small (<500 mw) unbound toxins with a low volume of distribution and minimal plasma protein binding (11), e.g., lithium, methanol, ethylene glycol, and salicylates. Continuous hemofiltration has been used in lithium toxicity (24), with better hemodynamic stability (25) but lower solute clearance than IHD.

The use of extracorporeal blood purification techniques in sepsis and septic shock is attractive but unproven. There were early observations of improved cardiovascular and respiratory function in patients with severe sepsis after commencement of continuous hemofiltration (26). This, together with the identification of inflammatory mediators in filtrate (27), led to efforts to increase inflammatory mediator removal during RRT. High-volume conventional hemofiltration (14, 28), large-pore hemofiltration (29), and plasma filtration with (30) or without (15) coupled adsorption have been examined in small clinical trials. There is currently no Level I evidence for the use of extracorporeal blood purification therapy in sepsis.

End-stage cardiac failure is characterized by progressive fluid retention, renal impairment, neurohumoral stimulation, and diuretic resistance (31). It was shown that patients with advanced cardiac failure can tolerate substantial fluid removal during ultrafiltration (12), with salutary effects that persist beyond the time of fluid removal. Improved renal function, decreased heart failure scores, lowered B natriuretic peptide levels, decreased hospital length of stay, and fewer readmissions have all been observed in case-controlled studies (32). Most recently, a small randomized controlled study showed that early ultrafiltration results in increased weight loss at 24 h compared with diuretics alone (33). Larger studies are warranted for this indication.

Cerebral edema can complicate IHD (34) and contribute to the clinical picture of disequilibrium. In patients with hepatic encephalopathy, early studies compared the effects of IHD and CRRT (35). CRRT was associated with less decrease in mean arterial pressure, less increase in intracranial pressure, and less change in cerebral perfusion pressure.

Choosing the Dose and Mode of RRT

Dialysis dose is a concept familiar to nephrologist in the setting of ESRF: Kt/V.

K is clearance (the volume of solute, usually urea, cleared in a given time), t is duration of treatment, and V is volume of distribution of the solute. Kt is the volume of plasma water cleared of solute during the session, and Kt/V is Kt as a proportion of its volume of distribution.

For example, a Kt/V of 1.0 for urea means that a total volume of plasma water equal to the volume of distribution of urea was cleared during the session. Using a single compartment exponential washout model, we can predict that the final concentration of the solute is approximately 37% of the starting concentration when the Kt/V is 1.0.

In chronic renal failure, a minimum Kt/V of 1.2 should be delivered three times per week (36). There has been one randomized controlled trial assessing dose of dialysis in ARF (7). Schiffl compared daily dialysis with alternate daily dialysis in 160 patients with ARF. The 28-day mortality using intention-to-treat analysis was 28% in the daily treated patients and 46% in the patients treated every other day. Multiple other outcomes were improved in the daily dialysis group. Although this trial was controversial (37), it suggests that dialysis every second day is insufficient in critically ill patients with ARF.

Quantification of clearance during CRRT can be likened to the calculation of creatinine clearance, which is described by the formula UV/P. U is the urine concentration of the solute, V is the volume collected in a given time, and P is the plasma concentration. During CRRT, if we know the volume of effluent produced in a given time and the concentration of solute (e.g., urea) in both effluent and plasma, we can calculate its clearance (38). The result is a value in milliliters per minute. To simplify the estimate further, let us assume that the sieving coefficient is 1.0, and that there is full concentration equilibrium between plasma water and dialysate. Then the effluent concentration will equal the plasma concentration, and clearance is simply equal to the rate of production of effluent from the hemofilter.

Ronco, in 2000 (39), randomized 425 critically ill patients with ARF to three different doses (ultrafiltration rates) of CRRT: 20, 35, or 45 mL/h/kg. Fifteen-day survivals were 41%, 57%, and 58%, respectively. This landmark study was one of the first to formally adjust dose of CRRT based on patient weight. Importantly, it suggests that there is a threshold minimum level of clearance required for adequate CRRT of approximately 35 mL/h/kg.

Debate regarding the relative merits of CRRT and IHD has continued for nearly 30 years. From the outset (5), the attraction of CRRT was its simplicity and cardiorespiratory stability compared with IHD. Now that CRRT is as complex as IHD

Prostacyclin

Prostaglandin (PG)-I$_2$ is a natural anticoagulant that is a potent antiplatelet agent and has been shown to reduce platelet microthrombi during dialysis. It is often used in patients with a high risk of bleeding, but because it is a potent arterial vasodilator, some patients develop symptomatic hypotension. It has been used on its own and in combination with low-dose heparin.

Other Anticoagulants

Heparinoids (e.g., danaparoid) have minimal effects on platelets and can be used in HITS (but remembering the potential cross reactivity in 5–10% of patients). However, standard markers of anticoagulation are not reliable and its effect is prolonged in renal failure. Factor Xa inhibitors (e.g., fondaparinux) and direct thrombin inhibitors (e.g., recombinant hirudin) can be safely used in HITS, but, to date, have limited use in CRRT.

Comment

A recent systematic review (16) found that there was no conclusive evidence to suggest one strategy over another, but the chosen method should take into account patient characteristics and local facilities. Heparin (UFN and LMWH) has the greatest evidence and experience behind it, but RCA is increasing in popularity and ease of use.

References

1. Kramer P, Wigger W, Rieger J, et al. Arteriovenous haemofiltration: a new and simple method for treatment of over-hydrated patients resistant to diuretics. *Klin Wochenschr.* 1977; 55: 1121–1122.
2. Palevsky PM. Dialysis Modality and Dosing Strategy in Acute Renal Failure. *Sem Dialysis.* 2006; 19: 165–170.
3. Van Biesen W, Vanholder R, Lameire N. Dialysis strategies in critically ill acute renal failure patients. *Curr Opin Crit Care.* 2003; 9: 491–495.
4. Palvesky PM, Baldwin I, Davenport A, et al. Renal replacement therapy and the kidney: minimising the impact of renal replacement therapy on recovery of acute renal failure. *Cur Opin Crit Care.* 2005; 11: 548–554.
5. Ricci Z, Ronco C, Bachetoni A, et al. Solute removal during continuous renal replacement therapy in critically ill patients; convection versus diffusion. *Crit Care.* 2006; 10: R67–R74.
6. Clark WR, Turk JE, Kraus MA, Gao D. Dose determinants in continuous renal replacement therapy. *Artif Organs.* 2003; 27: 815–820.
7. Ronco C, Bellomo R, Homal P, et al. Effects of different dose in continuous veno-venous haemofiltration on outcomes of acute renal failure: a prospective randomised trial. *Lancet.* 2000; 356: 26–30.
8. Bouman C, et al. Effects of early high-volume continuous Venovenous hemofiltratin of survival and recovery of renal function in intensive care patients with acute renal failure: a prospective randomized trial. *Crit Care Med.* 2000; 30: 2205–2211.
9. Saudan P, et al. Adding a dialysis dose to continuous hemofiltration increases survival in patients with acute renal failure. *Kidney Int.* 2006; 70: 1312–1317.
10. Cariou A, Vinsonneau C, Dhainaut JF. Adjunctive therapies in sepsis: an evidence-based review. *Crit Care Med.* 2004; 32: S562–S570.
11. www.adqi.net
12. Ronco C. Renal replacement therapy for acute kidney injury: let's follow the evidence. *Int J Artif Organs.* 2007; 30: 89–94.
13. Naka T, Bellomo R. Bench-to-bedside review: treating acid-base abnormalities in the intensive care unit–the role of renal replacement therapy. *Crit Care.* 2004; 8: 108–114.
14. Hilton PJ, Taylor J, Forni LG, Treacher DF. Bicarbonate-based haemofiltration in the management of acute renal failure with lactic acidosis. *QJM.* 1998; 4: 279–283.
15. Teehan GS, Liangos O, Lau J, et al. Dialysis membrane and modality in acute renal failure: understanding discordant meta-analyses. *Sem Dialysis.* 2003; 16: 356–360.
16. Oudemans-van Straaten HM, Wester JPJ, de Pont ACJM, Schetz MRC. Anticoagulation strategies in continuous renal replacement therapy: can the choice be evidence based? *Intensive Care Med.* 2006; 32: 188–202.

Suggested Reading

Bellomo R, Baldwin I, Ronco C, Golper T. *Atlas of Hemofiltration.* WB Saunders. 2002.

12
End-Stage Renal Disease

Emile Mohammed

There are now approximately one million people on renal replacement therapy worldwide. In the current era of chronic noncommunicable disease, this number is set to double within the next decade. Patients with end-stage renal disease (ESRD) carry a significantly higher cardiovascular morbidity and mortality compared with the general population. This is because of the "uremic" cardiovascular factors (Table 12.1). The result is that there will be a growing number of ESRD patients being managed within the intensive care unit (ICU) setting.

Hemodialysis and Peritoneal Dialysis

Mechanisms of Dialysis

There are two basic principles of dialysis that allow the body's homeostasis to be achieved in the absence of a natural kidney. They are as follows:

- Convection, in which there is movement (in large volumes) of solvent, which drags dissolved solute across a membrane with a hydrostatic pressure gradient.
- Diffusion, in which there is passive movement of solute from a high- to a low-concentration gradient across a membrane (Figure 12.1). Diffusion depends not only on the transmembrane gradient but the membrane characteristics (e.g., pore size).

Diffusion is more effective in clearing small molecules and convection improves mid-size molecule clearance.

Hemodialysis

Many hemodialysis (HD) techniques have been developed, particularly in the ICU setting, ranging from conventional HD, high-flux HD, hemodiafiltration, and hemofiltration. These techniques simply use varying degrees of convection or diffusion. For example, hemofiltration is a convective treatment with good clearance of mid-size molecules but with poor small molecule clearance. The converse holds for conventional intermittent HD.

Peritoneal Dialysis

The peritoneum acts as a natural semipermeable membrane. Dissolved waste products and water pass from the blood, via the peritoneal capillaries, through the mesothelial cells and interstitium to the peritoneal dialysis (PD) fluid (PDF). This process is referred to as ultrafiltration (Figure 12.2). Water-soluble waste products pass down a concentration gradient that is generated by an osmotic gradient. This, in turn, is created by glucose or glucose polymers added to the PDF.

PD regimens are all based on repetitions of a basic cycle, which comprises inflow of PDF, a dwell time of the PDF within the peritoneal cavity, and then drainage. The various types of PD are all based on this principle. They include continuous ambulatory PD (CAPD), automated PD (APD), tidal PD, and intermittent PD. Typical regimes are illustrated in Figure 12.3.

TABLE 12.1. Cardiovascular risk factors in the uremic patient

Traditional coronary risk factors (The Framingham Study)	Uremic-related cardiovascular risk factors
Hypertension	Increased extracellular fluid volume
High levels of low-density lipoprotein	Calcification and high calcium/phosphate product
Low levels of high-density lipoprotein	Parathyroid hormone
Smoking	Anemia
Diabetes	Oxidant stress
Older age	Malnutrition
Male sex	Pulse pressure
White race	Triglycerides
Physical inactivity	Lipoprotein remnants
Menopause	Lipoprotein A
Left ventricular hypertrophy	Homocysteine
	Inflammation (C-reactive protein)
	Sleep disorders

Clinical Parameters

Much debate surrounds the "optimal" dialysis dose, although a minimal dialysis dose has been universally accepted. Within the context of thrice-weekly HD, there seems to be no added benefit of high-dose dialysis compared with the conventional dose of dialysis (the HEMO study) (1). Dialysis adequacy is measured by urea kinetic modeling (UKM) using the urea reduction ratio, or Kt/V, where K is the dialyzer urea clearance, t is the duration of dialysis, and V is the urea distribution volume. In a well-nourished stable HD patient, a Kt/V of 0.8 to 1.0 is the minimum acceptable threshold per dialysis session. The Adequacy

of Peritoneal Dialysis in Mexico (ADEMEX) study (2) again reveals the same controversy of defining the optimal dialysis dose in PD patients. In this study, there was a neutral effect on patient survival between a control group on conventional CAPD compared with a study group on a modified prescription, which achieved increased small solute clearance, measured by peritoneal creatinine clearance and peritoneal Kt/V.

There are no "fixed targets" that determine dialysis adequacy in the ICU setting. Dialysis dose and duration must be determined by balancing the clinical condition of the patient, while achieving as normal a physiological state as possible.

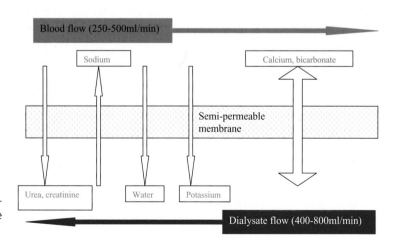

FIGURE 12.1. Diagrammatic representation of blood purification within the dialyzer.

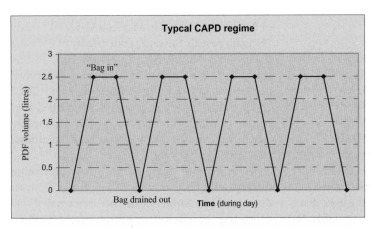

FIGURE 12.2. Ultrafiltration in PD.

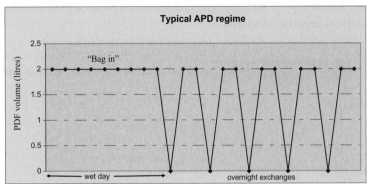

FIGURE 12.3. PD regimes.

The following clinical parameters act as guidelines to achieve this:

- *Target weight and blood pressure control.* Target weight is defined as the patient's weight in which all the fluid compartments are physiologically normal. Excess weight (which will be essentially salt and water) results in hypertension. The target weight is achieved by gradual weight reduction on successive dialyses until the patient is free from both pulmonary and peripheral edema, but, below which, hypotension occurs.
- *Acid-base balance.* Dialysis must be performed frequently and long enough to maintain normal acid-base balance.
- *Bone biochemistry.* Along with vitamin D supplementation, serum calcium and phosphate levels should be maintained within normal limits.
- *Nutritional state.* It is important to remember that a high proportion of ESRD patients within the ICU will have a low serum albumin, low body mass index, an inflammatory and/or hypercatabolic state, and a low dietary intake. It is, therefore, necessary to obtain dietary advice, treat correctable factors, give dietary supplements, and have a low threshold for nasogastric (NG), percutaneous endoscopic gastrostomy (PEG), or even parenteral nutrition, if indicated. Dialysis prescriptions must accommodate these nutritional requirements.

A good starting point for prescribing dialysis would be to continue the patient's regular dialysis regime and adjust the dose of dialysis, in conjunction with the nephrologists, to achieve the above parameters.

Dialysis-Related Complications

Hemodialysis

- *Hypotension.* Hypotension can be minimized with an accurate assessment of target weight, judicious use of antihypertensive medications, sodium restriction, increasing treatment duration, and careful choice of dialysis modality, e.g., hemodiafiltration in the cardiovascularly unstable patient.

- *Anaphylaxis.* Anaphylaxis can occur by complement activation with the use of a bioincompatible membrane and normally occurs within the first 20 minutes of treatment.
- *Catheter related-sepsis.* Catheter related-sepsis requires aggressive antibiotic treatment and catheter removal. If temporary catheters are being used, once weekly catheter changes are recommended.
- *Pyrogenic reactions.* Uncommon if ultrapure water is used.
- *Dialysis equilibrium syndrome.* Rare in established dialysis patients. It can occur from overaggressive dialysis causing a rapid reduction in serum osmolality and resulting in cerebral edema.
- Modern fail-safe machines minimize other complications such as *air embolism* and accidental circuit *disconnection*.

Peritoneal Dialysis

Although PD is a technically safe procedure, there may be clinical reasons to convert to temporary HD.

These are as follows:

- Abdominal surgery
- Diaphragmatic fluid leak resulting in effusions
- Respiratory compromise from splinting of diaphragm by PDF
- Severe hypoalbuminemic state
- Peritonitis or catheter-related sepsis
- Inadequate ultrafiltration in the context of aggressive fluid management and/or hypercatabolic state of the patient

Renal Transplantation

Renal transplantation represents the best mode of therapy for ESRD patients, both in cost effectiveness and quality of life (3). There have been many improvements in renal transplantation, such as the refinement of immunosuppression regimens, and patient-donor selection and work-up as well as their compatibilities. The major challenge facing transplantation is that its demand far outstrips the availability. Every effort should be made to increase the number of donors. In parallel to this, there is much research in the development of stem cell transplantation and xenotransplantation.

Evaluation, Selection, and Preparation of the Potential Transplant Recipient

General Evaluation

There are few absolute contraindications to renal transplantation. These are uncontrolled cancer, HIV positivity, active systemic infections, and/or any condition with a life expectancy of shorter than 2 years. Conditions increasing the risk of posttransplant morbidity and mortality include long duration of dialysis, previous incidence of recurrent infections, cardiovascular disease, and gastrointestinal complications. Such patients require a particularly careful work-up and aggressive management of risk factors (e.g., hypertension, obesity, and vascular disease) before transplantation.

Psychological Evaluation

The use of psychiatric screening is not universally adopted but may be useful in assessing compliance with immunosuppressive regimes. Poor compliance significantly worsens renal allograft outcomes.

Recurrent Renal Disease

It is important to ascertain the underlying cause of renal failure because some diseases recur in the transplanted kidney, most notably, focal and segmental glomerulosclerosis.

Immunological

ABO blood group must be compatible. HLA typing of donors and recipients allows assessment of compatibility. HLA DR is more important than HLA B, which is more important than HLA A. A lymphocyte cross-match is also performed: the recipient is screened for preexisting antibodies to donor lymphocytes, which arise in response to previous blood transfusions, pregnancies, or renal allografts. Such sensitization can cause severe hyperacute rejection.

Evaluation and Selection of Donors

There are two sources of donors:

Cadaveric: Cadaveric kidneys may be either from patients with brainstem death and a maintained cardiac output or from nonheart-beating donors. Donors with sepsis, malignancy, infection with hepatitis B, hepatitis C, HIV, or tuberculosis, or irreversible renal failure are not considered for donation.

Live: The use of kidneys from living donors is recommended for renal transplantation whenever possible, in light of the growing body of evidence of favorable outcomes after transplantation. Before being selected as a living donor, thorough counseling, medical, physical, and psychological evaluation is performed. Outcome studies have revealed lower mortality rates in living donors compared with the general population. This is probably caused in part by patient selection and the fact that this group of patients receive long-term medical follow-up.

Immunosuppression

The immunosuppression regime is tailored to each patient in an effort to minimize rejection as well as side effects. The following is a brief summary of drugs used, usually in combination. The commonest regime is triple therapy, e.g., cyclosporin, azathioprine, and prednisolone.

Corticosteroids have broad but potent immunosuppressive actions. They are used in high doses in induction therapy as well as for episodes of acute rejection. They are tapered to small maintenance doses or stopped completely over time. Because of the broad actions of corticosteroids, there are a large range of side effects.

Cyclosporin is a calcineurin inhibitor. Although there is little myelotoxicity, cyclosporin is nephrotoxic and does contribute to chronic allograft rejection. It is an important agent, because its introduction improved 1-year graft survival by 15 to 20%.

Tacrolimus is also a potent calcineurin inhibitor. Its side effect profile is similar to cyclosporin but seems to be more diabetogenic, particularly in the black population.

Azathioprine has been widely used for transplantation and it continues to be an integral part of many immunosuppression regimens. It inhibits purine metabolism and, therefore, cellular proliferation. There is a significant side-effect profile, most notably its myelosuppressive effect, which is worsened by concomitant use of other drugs such as allopurinol.

Mycophenolate mofetil acts similarly to azathioprine but is more specific for lymphocytes. Myelosuppression must also be monitored and mycophenolate mofetil has more gastrointestinal side effects than azathioprine.

Daclizumab and *basiliximab* are anti-CD25 antibodies. They target activated T cells only and are used as an induction agent to prevent early rejection.

Polyclonal antibodies to T-cells, ALG and ATG, as well as *monoclonal antibody to T cells*, OKT3, are used to treat refractory acute rejection and sometimes used as an induction agent to prevent rejection. These drugs are used cautiously because their administration is associated with cytokine release syndrome and pulmonary edema. Other side effects include subsequent infection and posttransplantation lymphoproliferative disease (PTLD).

Complications of Transplantation

Immediate

- *Acute tubular necrosis* is the commonest cause of early graft function and is more likely to occur with prolonged ischemic times and asystolic, hypotensive, or elderly donors.
- *Surgical complications* are now the commonest cause of early graft loss. These include renal vein and arterial thrombosis and urinary leaks. These complications are surveyed for with Doppler ultrasound and isotope scanning. Occasionally renal angiography or surgical reexploration is required in the anuric kidney.
- *Hyperacute rejection* is now very uncommon, with the more meticulous screening for the presence of preexisting antibodies. The only available treatment is graft nephrectomy.

Early

- *Acute rejection* should be suspected in patients with established graft function who then experience a rise in serum creatinine. A biopsy is usually required to confirm the clinical diagnosis and the treatment involves high-dose steroids, usually with some modification of the immunosuppression regime. Antibodies are considered in steroid-refractory acute rejection.
- *Infectious complications* tend to vary with time after transplantation. Within the first month after transplantation, most infections are surgically related, such as atelectasis and wound infection. From 1 to 6 months after transplantation, opportunistic infections can emerge, such as *Pneumocystis carinii* and *Aspergillus fumigatus*. Clinical infection caused by the effects of modulating viruses, cytomegalovirus (CMV) and Epstein-Barr virus (EBV) are serious complications for which there should be surveillance with prophylaxis administered where appropriate. PTLD in the early period tends to be an EBV-related malignancy.
- *Mechanical complications*, such as arterial and ureteric stenoses and lymphoceles exerting local pressure, sometimes evolve as a cause of deteriorating graft function.

Late

- *Chronic rejection* occurs secondary to a combination of immunological and nonimmunological factors. The result is an irreversible progressive decline in graft function and is often associated with proteinuria.
- *Recurrence of original disease* may result in graft failure. There is a particularly high rate of recurrence of focal and segmental glomerulosclerosis but it is difficult to predict and, therefore, is not a contraindication to transplantation.
- *Cardiovascular disease* is the main cause of death in the transplant population and the rate of cardiovascular disease is higher than in the general population. This is because of the additional risk factors of the ESRD population (Table 12.1) as well as the adverse effects of the immunosuppressive agents.
- *Malignancy*, in particular, skin cancer, is three times more common than the general population.

Other cancers that should be screened for include renal, cervical, and vaginal cancers.

Summary

ESRD and its complications are becoming more commonplace, particularly in the ICU environment. The challenges associated with this group of patients also continue to rise and requires a multidisciplinary approach, which includes the intensivist and the nephrologist.

References

1. Eknoyan G, Beck GJ, Cheung AK, et al. Hemodialysis (HEMO) Study Group. Effect of dialysis dose and membrane flux in maintenance hemodialysis. *N Engl J Med* 2002; 347(25): 2010–2019.
2. Paniagua R, Amato D, Vonesh E, et al. Health-related quality of life predicts outcomes but is not affected by peritoneal clearance: The ADEMEX trial. *Kidney Int* 2005; 67(3): 1093–1104.
3. The EBPG Expert Group on Renal Transplantation. European Best Practice Guidelines for Renal Transplantation (Part 1). *Nephrol Dial Transplant* 2000; 15(Supp 7): 1–85.

Suggested Reading

Davison AM, Cameron S, Grunfeld J-P, et al. Oxford Textbook of Clinical Nephrology. 3rd edition. Oxford: Oxford University Press. 2005.
Levy J, Brown E, Morgan J. Oxford Handbook of Dialysis. Oxford: Oxford University Press. 2001.

TABLE 15.3. Clinical effects of metabolic acidosis and metabolic alkalosis

	Metabolic acidosis	Metabolic alkalosis
Cardiac	• Reduced myocardial contractility and cardiac failure (*but unclear association in clinical practice*) • Resistance to catecholamines • Increased risk of arrhythmias	• Decreased myocardial perfusion caused by arteriolar constriction • Reduced angina threshold • Increased risk of arrhythmias
Respiratory	• Stimulation of the carotid body and aortic chemoreceptors causing hyperventilation (*Kussmaul respiration*)	• Depressed ventilation (*causing compensatory respiratory acidosis*), which could lead to failure to wean a patient from mechanical ventilation
Neurological	• Impaired consciousness (*mechanism not fully understood and not clearly correlating with the degree of acidosis*) • Intracerebral vasodilation (*may be clinically significant in the setting of already raised intracranial pressure*)	• Decreased cerebral blood flow caused by arteriolar constriction • Headache, confusion, mental obtundation • Neuromuscular excitability: seizures and tetany (*related to reduction in ionized calcium level*)
Metabolic and immune	• Hyperkalemia (*extracellular potassium shifts*) • Glucose intolerance (*inhibition of glycolysis and hepatic gluconeogenesis*) • Immune activation	• Hypokalemia • Hypomagnesemia • Hypophosphatemia • Stimulation of aerobic glycolysis leading production of lactic acid and ketoacids • Decreased plasma ionized calcium concentration

Note: the effects of severe alkalemia (pH > 7.60) appear more pronounced with respiratory rather than metabolic alkalosis.

Equation 15.3:

$$SIDa - SIDe = SIG \text{ (equals zero unless unmeasured anions or cations present)}$$

By using this approach, a change in the balance between strong anions and cations accounts for acid-base disturbances seen on the ICU. For example, *excess* chloride from a high-volume saline infusion reduces the SID, causing an acidosis. A *loss* of chloride from a large nasogastric output increases the SID, causing an alkalosis.

The modern debate now centers on which is the best and most practical method of assessing acid-base disorders in critically ill patients, and, in particular, detecting the presence of unmeasured anions: the SIG. To date, neither the SIG, corrected AG, or corrected SBE has been found to be overwhelmingly superior to the other, but all have been found to be predictors of increased mortality (10, 11).

Lactic Acidosis (Table 15.4)

When more lactate is produced than is metabolized, hyperlactatemia occurs. Elevated levels are generally taken to indicate anaerobic metabolism caused by generalized or regional tissue hypoxia (12). However, it is important to remember that lactate can be produced under aerobic conditions, especially in the setting of inflammatory processes. In sepsis, inflammatory mediators can accelerate aerobic glycolysis, leading to increased glucose turnover and increased lactate production (12, 13). Specific organs are also capable of producing excess lactate under times of stress, for example, the lungs and gut (12, 13).

Elevated lactate levels may also indicate decreased clearance (12). Lactate is mostly metabolized by the liver (50%), and decreased clearance can occur with impaired liver function or decreased liver blood flow.

Unless lactate levels are specifically measured, an elevated level may be "missed" by the AG or SBE because of factors such as hypoalbuminemia. In addition, hyperlactatemia is not always accompanied by an acidosis.

Elevated lactate levels, particularly those that fail to clear during the first 24 hours, have been repeatedly shown to correlate with a poor outcome (11, 14, 15).

Use of Sodium Bicarbonate

Controversy exists regarding the use of alkali therapy (e.g., sodium bicarbonate) to treat metabolic acidosis (16). No clinical studies have shown

TABLE 15.4. Classification of lactic acidosis

Type A (hypoxic)
   Circulatory insufficiency (e.g., shock, cardiac arrest)
   Regional hypoperfusion
   Carbon monoxide and cyanide poisoning (caused by mitochondrial enzyme inhibition)
   Severe hypoxia
   Severe exercise/prolonged seizures (caused by increased muscle activity)
   Severe anemia

Type B (nonhypoxic)
   Sepsis in general (caused by accelerated aerobic glycolysis and mitochondrial dysfunction) and with specific infections (e.g., cholera, falciparum malaria, AIDS)
   Thiamine deficiency (thiamine is a cofactor of pyruvate dehydrogenase)
   Fulminant hepatic failure, severe liver disease
   Alcoholism (ethanol oxidation increases the conversion of pyruvate to lactate and inhibits of pathways of pyruvate metabolism)
   Severe renal failure
   Malignancy, leukemia, and lymphoma
   Short bowel syndrome (D lactic acidosis)
   Diabetic ketoacidosis (ketones may inhibit hepatic lactate uptake)

Type B: drug induced
   Phenformin/metformin
   Ethanol, methanol, ethylene glycol
   Salicylate poisoning
   Paracetamol poisoning
   Intravenous fructose, sorbitol
   Cyanide
   β-agonists (e.g., salbutamol, adrenaline, caused by increased glyconeogenesis, glycogenolysis, lipolysis, and cyclic AMP activity)

Type B: inborn errors of metabolism
   Glucose 6 phosphatase deficiency
   Fructose 1,6 diphosphatase deficiency
   Deficiency of enzymes of oxidative phosphorylation

a benefit on outcome in patients with lactic acidosis, but it is difficult to separate the effects of the acidosis from the effects of the underlying pathological condition.

Sodium bicarbonate is not without risks, including:

- Acute fluid overload.
- Alkaline "overshoot" caused by subsequent metabolism of organic salts increasing the bicarbonate concentration.
- Paradoxical intracellular acidosis. CO_2 released diffuses more quickly than bicarbonate ions into cells, therefore, initially lowering the intracellular pH. *There is debate regarding whether this is clinically significant.*

Use of Renal Replacement Therapy

In acute renal failure, the daily production of mineral acids is adequately matched by the effi-

cacy of renal replacement therapy (RRT) techniques, therefore, the acidosis can be cleared within 48 hours (16). Despite the fact that lactate has a low molecular weight and it is easily removed by continuous therapies, RRT has been shown to contribute to only less than 3% of total lactate clearance (17). It may be that RRT plays a role in improving the overall clinical situation (e.g., hemodynamic and fluid status), therefore, promoting the clearance of lactate, rather than actually removing it.

Metabolic Alkalosis

Metabolic alkalosis is common, but carries an associated mortality that increases with increasing pH, especially pH higher than 7.55 (18). The cause, rather than the alkalosis itself, may be the reason for the increased mortality.

Metabolic alkalosis can be classified clinically (Table 15.2) or according to the underlying pathophysiology: initiating process or perpetuating processes (18).

Initiating Processes

1. *Loss of hydrogen ions* through the kidney (e.g., loop diuretics, primary hyperaldosteronism) or gastrointestinal tract (e.g., vomiting, nasogastric suctioning).
2. *Accumulation of alkali* from exogenous (e.g., sodium bicarbonate in the setting of renal insufficiency) or endogenous sources (e.g., metabolism of ketones after diabetic ketoacidosis).

The kidneys have a large capacity to excrete excess bicarbonate and are mostly able to correct the alkalosis; however, in certain situations, the kidney will *retain* rather than excrete alkali, therefore, *perpetuating* the alkalosis. The persistence of a metabolic alkalosis suggests there is an ongoing, untreated process.

Perpetuating Factors

1. *Hypovolemia.* Decreased renal perfusion stimulates the renin-angiotensin-aldosterone system (RAAS), therefore, increasing sodium absorption and hydrogen ion secretion.
2. *Chloride depletion.* Stimulation of the RAAS leads to increased bicarbonate reabsorption in the absence of adequate chloride.
3. *Severe hypokalemia.* Caused by an intracellular shift of hydrogen ions in exchange for potassium.
4. *Reduced glomerular filtration rate* (GFR). Reduction in GFR causes a decrease in filtered bicarbonate.

Treatment

1. Correct the primary cause if possible, e.g., stop or reduce diuretics.
2. Address perpetuating factors. Most forms of metabolic alkalosis are chloride responsive, and isotonic sodium chloride will correct both chloride and volume depletion. As the chloride deficit is corrected, there will be an alkaline diuresis and the plasma bicarbonate will start to normalize.

3. Consider specific treatments, e.g., surgery for an adrenal adenoma or spironolactone for hyperaldosteronism.
4. Other:
   a. Hydrochloric acid: rarely used.
   b. Acetazolamide: increases bicarbonate loss, but only if GFR is adequate.
   c. RRT: in patients with severe cardiac or renal disease, RRT may assist volume and electrolyte correction. Standard replacement fluids will need modification as they contain bicarbonate or its precursor lactate.

References

1. Stewart PA. Modern quantitative acid-base chemistry. *Can J Pharmacol.* 1983; 61: 1444–1461.
2. Story DA. Bench-to-bedside review: A brief history of clinical acid-base. *Crit Care.* 2004; 8: 253–258.
3. Kellum JA. Determinants of blood pH in health and disease. *Crit Care.* 2000; 4: 6–14.
4. Kaplan LJ, Frangos S. Clinical review: Acid-base abnormalities in the intensive care unit. *Crit Care.* 2005; 9: 198–203.
5. Morgan TJ. Clinical review: The meaning of acid-base abnormalities in the intensive care unit—effects of fluid administration. *Crit Care.* 2005; 9: 204–211.
6. Morgan TJ. What exactly is the strong ion gap, and does anybody care? *Crit Care Resusc.* 2004; 6: 155–166.
7. Figge J, Jabor A, Kazda A, Fencl V. Anion gap and hypoproteinaemia. *Crit Care Med.* 1998; 26: 1807–1810.
8. Fencl V, Jabor A, Kazda A, Figge J. Diagnosis of metabolic acid-base disturbances in critically ill patients. *Am J Resp Crit Care Med.* 2000; 162: 2246–2251.
9. Story DA, Poustie S, Bellomo R. Estimating unmeasured anions in critically ill patients: anion gap, base deficit and strong ion gap. *Anaesthesia.* 2002; 57: 1102–1133.
10. Kaplan LJ, Kellum JA. Initial pH, base deficit, lactate, anion gap, strong ion difference, and strong ion gap predict outcome from major vascular injury. *Crit Care Med.* 2004; 32: 1120–1124.
11. Smith I, Kumar P, Molloy S, et al. Base excess and lactate as prognostic indicators for patients admitted to intensive care. *Intensive Care Med.* 2001; 27: 74–83.
12. De Backer D. Lactic acidosis. *Intensive Care Med.* 2003; 29: 699–702.

13. Bellomo R, Ronco C. The pathogenesis of lactic acidosis in sepsis. *Curr Opin Crit Care.* 1999; 5: 452–457.

14. Stacpoole PW, Wright EC, Baumgartner TG, et al. for the DCA-Lactic acidosis Study Group: Natural history and course of acquired lactic acidosis in adults. *Am J Med.* 1994; 97: 47–54.

15. Husain FA, Martin MJ, Mullenix PS, et al. Serum lactate and base deficit as predictors of mortality and morbidity. *Am J Surg.* 2003; 185(5): 485–491.

16. Levraut J, Grimaud D. Treatment of metabolic acidosis. *Curr Opin Crit Care.* 2003; 9: 260–265.

17. Levraut J, Ciebiera JP, Jambou P, et al. Effect of continuous venovenous hemofiltration with dialysis on lactate clearance in critically ill patients. *Crit Care Med.* 1997; 25(1): 58–62.

18. Galla JH. Metabolic alkalosis. *J Am Soc Nephrol.* 2000; 11: 369–375.

Index